QUICK BACKACHE RELIEF WITHOUT DRUGS

Howard Kurland, M.D.

ORBIS PUBLISHING LIMITED · LONDON

This edition published by Orbis Publishing Limited 1982

Printed in Great Britain by Butler & Tanner Ltd, Frome and London

ISBN: 0-85613-407-4

CONTENTS

Prologue
SOME INTRODUCTORY ADVICE

This book contains much wisdom about how to relieve backache. It may teach you how you can live with backache without taking drugs. The techniques described in this book can enable you to produce acupuncture-like effects in your own body. You can learn to do so by yourself and without the use of needles or gadgets.

Oriental acupuncturists have achieved pain relief for thousands of years. Studies supported by the United States National Institutes of Health have recently documented the scientific validity of such effects.

When I developed the techniques of auto-acupressure, I did not have the comfort of scientific documentation for such drugless pain relief. However, both personal experience and observation of many patients have convinced me that these techniques are truly effective. You will clearly understand how I personally used these techniques to restore my own functioning when you read about 'My Back'.

Chapter 1
MY BACK

An eerie premonition of danger haunted me throughout the month. It was the middle 1960s and I was a medical officer in the United States Navy. Attending a medical meeting at the University of California should not have been a menacing thought. Nevertheless, a mysterious sense of dread appeared every time I considered it. When the time of the seminar finally arrived, I overcame my foreboding and drove toward the meeting. I was never able to attend it.

The impact occurred as my car waited at the rear of a line of traffic on a highway in San Francisco. The police report stated that the car which struck me from behind was travelling at sixty-five miles per hour. My car was sent hurtling on the shoulder of an elevated freeway. The locked-brake skid lasted more than sixty feet. I instinctively clung to the steering wheel, terrified that the car would go over the edge. That encounter with terror remained frozen into my mind for hours afterwards. It numbed the awareness of traumatic injuries that my body had suffered.

The morning after the accident, I awoke with my lower back hurting so severely that I could hardly stand up. Sitting was particularly painful. The pain travelled down my right leg. When I tried to walk, I felt a sharp new spear of pain every time I moved that leg forward.

An orthopaedic surgeon determined that the car accident had damaged my back. It appeared that there was an injury to one of the discs in the low back area. We will study the intervertebral discs in more detail later, for they are at the root of many of the most intractable back problems. It is enough to say for now that they are pads of tough, resilient tissue that separate the bones of the spine.

For six months I required physical therapy. It included heat treatments, massage, and ultrasonic therapy. After that time, I was able to carry on my normal life again. I had to be careful, of course. My back would hurt sometimes. I had to avoid sitting in soft chairs or in a slumped position. I also had to sleep on a firm mattress at night. But aside from these and a few other precautionary measures, my low back ceased to cause me any significant trouble.

I was not careful enough. Several years after the car accident that started it all, I injured my back again. It happened this time when I was trying to lift a hundred pound sack of garden fertilizer from the boot of my car. It was almost impossible to accomplish this feat correctly. There was no way to get my legs under the weight. The design of the boot almost required me to lift in a way that put maximum strain on my back. I bent forward, with the car's rear bumper against my knees and thighs. I lifted by pulling with my back muscles alone. Since my back had a previously weakened area, it was prone to injury.

Before I had that sack of fertilizer halfway out of the boot, a spasm of excruciating pain gripped my lower back and radiated down my right leg. I had injured an intervertebral disc. In the years since the car accident, my back had healed and strengthened enough to withstand ordinary demands. But it had not become strong enough to take that exaggerated abuse.

The injury was significant: I needed complete bed rest for two weeks. My doctor prescribed pain-killing drugs. He also prescribed muscle relaxants to relieve the muscular spasm that is often an important secondary cause of backache. When I was finally allowed to move about, I had to wear an orthopaedic brace. This device was designed, in effect, to take part of my upper-body weight off my spine and rest it on my hips. It was awkward and uncomfortable, but it did allow the healing process to take place. In time, I was able to stand and walk without the brace. My condition improved gradually. I was more careful than before. As long as I was aware of my back's limitations, I found I was able to live a full, active life.

Then, around 1970, I encountered more trouble. It was even more serious. I had been scuba diving with a group off Palancar Reef near Cozumel, Mexico. Returning from a deep dive, more than 100 feet below the surface, we found that the ocean began to grow rougher than we or our diving guides liked. Several less experienced divers panicked in the choppy surf and needed help to board the boat. Struggling to hold my position in an increasingly rough ocean, I had to spend about half an hour waiting to board. By the time my turn came to climb up the ladder, I was utterly exhausted.

My upper body and scuba gear felt weightless in the water. But as I hauled myself up the ladder, all that weight suddenly rested on my spine. As I put my foot on the second rung and started to lift, I felt an indescribably agonizing stab of pain. It was like a high-voltage electric shock going down my right leg.

The orthopaedic examination revealed the weakened intervertebral disc had herniated. For medical reasons that are not relevant here, surgery was considered inadvisable. The best my doctor could do was return me to near-normal living with my back as it was.

The months that followed were among the least pleasant of my life. I spent the first week under heavy medication, in bed and in traction. When I was finally allowed out of bed, a specialist put me into a form-fitting brace that held my back virtually rigid. This brace allowed me to get around, but just barely.

I could walk on a level surface without great pain as long as I moved cautiously, but that was about all. Merely stepping off a low kerb caused agony. I could not carry my briefcase; the added weight on one side, even a light weight, put more strain on my injured spine than it could handle. What troubled me most of all was that the injury hampered my ability to work at my profession. I was then, as now, a neurologist. Part of a neurologist's work involves testing patients' muscular strength and responsiveness. To do this, the neurologist must push and pull against the patient in various ways. My injured back would not allow me to do this.

I had to spend many weekends in bed, sometimes in traction. My back needed that much rest if it was going to function at all during the week.

From the beginning, I had tried to avoid taking pain-killing drugs because my medical practice required me to be alert. In any case, I did not want to become dependent on drugs, trapped in a life-style of swallowing pills to help me struggle through each day. Instead of getting addicted to drugs, I became addicted to my brace. It was unwieldy and uncomfortable. It made my ribs ache, caused pain and muscle spasm in my shoulders, but I was afraid to walk around without it.

I wore it for more than a year. All during that time, I realized perfectly well what was happening. I knew I was growing more dependent on the brace than was good for me. I knew I would have to get rid of it sometime, somehow, or I might condemn myself to wearing it for life. Now that the healing process was well begun, my back needed a chance to strengthen itself so that it would return to something like its normal functioning. As long as I wore the brace, no such strengthening could happen.

Yet, I knew there would be a lot of pain when I took the brace off; pain that might last for months, even years. As any backache sufferer knows, this kind of pain cannot be easily shrugged off. How would I carry on my profession and the rest of my life under such conditions? There seemed to be only one answer: to keep myself drugged with pain-killers. But that was an answer I had already rejected.

Was there no way out?

I had been casually interested in acupuncture for many years. I had never really studied it or considered it seriously as a bona fide approach to healing or pain relief. Like the majority of Western doctors, I was highly sceptical about its alleged effectiveness. My attitude towards it was one of amused tolerance: it was a type of Oriental mysticism, and if people wanted to play around with it, I did not begrudge them their fun. But if they expected that a visit to an acupuncturist would bring tangible improvements in their medical problems, they were probably wasting their money.

That was what I thought.

A friend in Hong Kong had spent a good deal of time trying to convince me of the merits of acupuncture. During one of my visits with him, as we sailed around Hong Kong's harbour in his boat, he cited case histories of acupuncture patients whose ailments had been successfully treated. Many of these stories were highly dramatic. I might have tried to argue that they were exaggerated or untrue, but I had no reason to think my friend would deliberately try to deceive me. I was willing to grant that the stories might be strictly and literally true. Or at least that my friend was telling the truth as he had seen it, heard it, and interpreted it. Even so, I remained sceptical.

For, as I pointed out to my friend, there could be more than one way to interpret a situation in which an alleged medical treatment produces an apparent cure of an asserted ailment.

One possibility: the ailment never existed except in the patient's imagination. In this kind of situation, an apparent 'cure' might be effected by any procedure the patient believes in, even by a sugar pill, as long as the patient is convinced it is a miracle drug. The procedure or pill might seem to work for this one patient. As far as the patient is concerned, it actually *does* work; but this does not mean it can be expected to work for anybody else.

Another possibility: the ailment was invented by the acupuncturist. This is one of the oldest tricks in the history of medical quackery, and I have never doubted that it is practised in the Orient as often as in the West. It works like this: a patient goes to a self-styled 'doctor' with vague complaints of listlessness, fatigue, loss of sexual vigour, and so on. The doctor convinces the patient that these are symptoms of some serious-sounding disease for which he, the doctor, knows just the treatment. The treatment is, of course, expensive and of years-long duration. It is medically worthless. However, as an adjunct to the treatment, the doctor counsels the patient to improve his diet, get more exercise, stop smoking, and so on. The patient's vigour returns, and he goes away believing he has been miraculously cured.

Another possibility: the ailment was real, but it was already being alleviated by natural processes. The patient would have got better whether he visited an acupuncturist or not. He now credits acupuncture for an outcome that was actually brought about by his body's own natural defences and repair mechanisms.

Thus, as I told my friend, it would take more than a collection of dramatic case stories to convince me that acupuncture was a genuinely useful medical procedure.

Then came the scuba-diving episode, the brace, and the drugs. I was desperate for a way out of the dilemma, willing to try anything that offered even the faintest promise. When a chance arose for me to take another trip to the Orient, I resolved to give acupuncture a try.

I had heard many claims for acupuncture, as I have said, not only from my Hong Kong friend but also from other people. Prominent among these claims was the assertion that acupuncture is particularly useful in controlling chronic pain. There are many kinds of pain whose causes, for various reasons, do not lend themselves to a safe, practical treatment. In such situations the indicated procedure is to treat the pain symptom itself. Common types of headache fall into this category, and so do many kinds of backache.

I did not really believe acupuncture could do anything to relieve pain, especially pain as severe as that which I was experiencing in my lower back. However, I resolved to keep an open mind on the subject. I travelled to Taipei. With an English-speaking Chinese nurse as interpreter, I visited several acupuncturists, watched their techniques, asked questions. Finally I gathered enough courage to submit to a treatment.

The clinic I chose for this first treatment was, like most others I had seen in Taipei, astoundingly dirty. As a Western physician, I had had it drummed into me since my days as a medical student that good medicine starts with conditions of antiseptic cleanliness. Looking around at the acupuncturist's dusty rooms with their grimy, fly-specked walls, I found all my doubts increasing. How could any worthwhile medicine be practised in an environment like this?

But I stuck with my original decision: I would go through with this one treatment, keep my mind open, and judge the acupuncturist by his final results. If he proved his skill with his needle, I would forgive him for neglecting his broom and scrubbing brush.

As I lay down on his dirty treatment table, my back and leg were throbbing painfully. I had not worn my brace that day. Moreover, the clinic was on the second floor of a building, and the climb up the stairs had thrown my back muscles into spasm. My back hurt quite severely, but I was determined to give the acupuncturist a thorough test.

He inserted needles at several points in my back and shoulders.

And my pain abruptly vanished.

I was astonished. I kept thinking, This can't be true! But it was patently true. My back muscles were comfortably relaxed, and the pain that I should have felt, had quite confidently expected to feel, simply was not there.

That was how I became a student, and eventually a practitioner, of acupuncture. I visited many other acupuncturists in Taiwan, Hong Kong, and Japan; then went on studying the technique when I returned home. Since it is difficult and sometimes unpleasant to insert needles in oneself, I paid particular attention to an alternative technique that the Chinese call *finger needle*. This means using the fingernails or thumbnails instead of a needle. Because I did not have an experienced acupuncturist to treat me, I had to become adept at relieving my back pain by pressing certain body points with my thumbnails. I found that I could alleviate the pain instantly, at the moment a spasm began, by stopping whatever I was doing and applying pressure for a short time. There was no longer any reason to fear the pain. I discarded my brace and my pain medicines.

I went back to the Orient about a year later, hoping

to find answers to some questions that had arisen during my studies of acupuncture techniques. I found that many of my acupuncturist friends were excited by *auricular* therapy, the use of needle or pressure points on the ears. It was not a new technique; it was being resurrected after having been ignored for a century or more. It was being grounded in modern anatomy and physiology with innovative work begun by a French neurophysiologist named Nogier. His discoveries were rapidly absorbed in China.

I was enormously sceptical at first. But then I tried it on myself and was amazed by its effectiveness in relieving back pain. Specific areas on the ear, I learned, reflect the entire body in miniature. I developed an ear point system of auto-acupressure. I will teach you how to use both ear point and body point systems to control the pain in your back.

Not long after I returned from that trip to the Orient, I gained firsthand knowledge of the effectiveness of ear point auto-acupressure. I was injured again. An unlicensed fourteen-year-old driver spun his car out of control. I had been riding a bicycle next to a high kerb. When the car struck, I was thrown through the air. My back shattered landing on the concrete road. The accident reinjured the same disc that had given me so much trouble before.

After that scuba-diving episode a few years back, I had thought I was experiencing backache at its worst. I was terribly wrong. The pain at that time had indeed been intense, but it seemed almost trivial to me in the months after the car-and-bike accident. In this latest accident, I had sustained injuries not only to my low back, but also severe injuries to my neck. For weeks, I was in such intense pain that I could not sleep at night without using the drugs which my orthopaedist had prescribed.

Perhaps it surprises you that I went back to using drugs, and that I openly admit it in this book. But there is a serious purpose behind this admission. I am a scientist, not a sideshow pitchman. My intent is to tell you precisely what auto-acupressure can and cannot do. I want you to learn how to use it, and develop confidence in its pain-relieving effects. If I were to oversell it, claiming miracles that could never happen, I would only defeat my own purpose.

I kept my intake of all medications to a minimum. While using prescribed pain relievers and muscle relaxants to help me sleep, I took none of those drugs in waking hours. Instead, I used to control the pain and muscle spasm with ear point and body point acupressure. The only medication I took in the daytime was the short course of anti-inflammatory agents my orthopaedist advised.

Within two months, I was able to stop taking medication for my back altogether. My orthopaedic doctor advised me to use both a back brace and a neck brace. However, I was soon able to discard those also. Auto-acupressure, especially ear point auto-acupressure, helped me back to a normal life.

And that is the story of my back. I have told the story to establish my credentials with you. When I talk about pain, I think you will have to grant that I know my subject intimately.

Chapter 2
OUR BACKS

Backache, particularly in the lower or lumbar region, is among the most common scourges of mankind. The US National Center for Health Statistics says that people visit doctors with this complaint more than with any other, except respiratory infections. Some industrial companies report that backache is the number one cause of absenteeism: it causes more work time to be lost than does any other kind of ailment, *including* respiratory infections.

Very few people are immune. One commonly accepted estimate is that four out of every five adults, at some time in their lives, will experience backaches that are severe enough to interfere appreciably with normal daily living. Some of these people are relatively lucky: their backaches do not come often or last long. But about a third will find, eventually, that their backaches recur often enough and last long enough to be called chronic.

The human back is a remarkable structure of bone, muscle, ligament, and other tissues. It is strong but often not quite strong enough for the punishment it is required to absorb. As we will see later in the book, some scientists hold that it is innately weak, while others feel it would be strong enough to do its job if the average man and woman treated it with greater care. Whatever the truth of this debate may be, the central fact is that backaches are among humanity's most widespread ailments. No other part of the body's skeletal structure causes trouble so often.

Is there any escape from this suffering? In a very small percentage of cases, breakdowns of the back can be wholly or partially repaired with surgery. But in the vast majority of cases, surgery is not advisable or is not practical. Most backache sufferers must content themselves with trying to control the pain and muscle spasm with drugs.

According to the American Food and Drug Administration, more varieties of over-the-counter pills and liniments and other medications are sold for relief of backache than for any other ailment, including headaches and the common cold. There is enormous consumption of analgesics or pain-deadeners. Many are based on aspirin (acetylsalicylic acid), which is produced in the USA at a rate of 15,000 tons a year: up to 50 tons *a day* in some months. For people who cannot take aspirin because of stomach upset or other problems, there are analgesics based on chemicals other than aspirin. Then there are various medicines that claim to relieve backaches by improving the function of the liver, kidneys, bowels and so on. Malfunctions of these and other organs are thought to cause backache in some people. Finally there are large numbers of rub-on-the-skin medications. They purportedly alleviate backache and muscle spasm by producing beneficial heat in the affected area.

In addition to medications such as these, backache sufferers are invited to buy all kinds of gadgetry and hardware. The list is long: trusses, braces, heating pads, orthopaedic mattresses, bedboards, electrical massage gadgets, special shoes that allegedly improve the posture, whirlpool baths, and so on.

Some of these non-prescription drugs and gadgets work tolerably well for some people, but they fail to give lasting relief for most. And even a relatively mild drug such as aspirin can be highly dangerous to certain people when taken over a long span of time.

If the sufferer fails to get relief from over-the-counter drugs and gadgetry, he or she may seek help from a medical doctor. The doctor may prescribe stronger pain-deadening or muscle-relaxing drugs. But these may be even more dangerous than the over-the-counter remedies.

Or perhaps the sufferer goes to a chiropractor. Though the British and American Medical Associations have refused to endorse chiropractic as a worthwhile medical technique, it is not my intention in this book to pick a fight with chiropractors. I will only comment that some people say their backs feel better after a chiropractic manipulation, while others say they get only short-term relief or no relief. Forceful manipulation of certain back disorders, which we will discuss in Chapter 5, might result in serious injury to the spinal column, with the possibility of permanent paralysis.

The vast majority of sufferers seem to go through roughly the same history. At first there is a period of desperate experimentation. The sufferer tries all kinds of peculiar medicines, gadgets, treatments, and self-help techniques. Finally, when these fail, he or she falls back on drugs: prescription analgesics and muscle relaxants, over-the-counter remedies, or combinations of these.

The potential hazards of such drugs are enormous. Let us, therefore, reflect on some questions:

Do you like the idea of a drug-dominated life? A life in which you must take drugs that dull or distort your intellect? Do you want to take unnecessary drugs? *Especially when you suspect or know those drugs are doing serious damage in your body?*

Until now, most backache sufferers have had to answer those questions in a spirit of unhappy resignation: 'No, I don't like the idea of a drug-taking life-style. I don't like it at all. But what else can I do? It's either the drugs or the pain.'

This book offers you a way out of this apparent trap. It is medically sound, effective, safe, inexpensive, and utterly practical.

I call it *auto-acupressure*. In a preceding book, I described the use of this technique in treating headaches. This book details the results of my further studies into the problem of relieving backaches. As you recall from Chapter 1, it is a problem with which I am personally, painfully familiar.

Auto-acupressure is derived from and related to *acupuncture*, an Oriental medical technique in which pain and other problems are treated by inserting and manipulating needles at certain carefully chosen body points. Acupuncture is a technique that demonstrably works (although it has been oversold and has often fallen into the hands of blunderers and quacks). However, a drawback of acupuncture is that it does not lend itself readily to self-treatment.

There are some people who can insert and manipulate acupuncture needles in themselves without qualms, who feel comfortable doing so, and who achieve good results. But they are a tiny minority, and to do so, in my opinion, is dangerous. That is why I developed my system of auto-acupressure. No needles are involved in this technique. You use only your fingers and thumbnails. When you grow efficient with the technique, the results are similar to those that a professional acupuncturist would obtain with a needle.

This book will present everything you need to know to control backache and muscle spasm with auto-acupressure. I am offering you a double reward that may be among the most valuable you have ever received in your life: *relative freedom from severe and/or prolonged backache, and relative freedom from drugs.*

I called it a reward. Properly speaking, a reward is earned. To make the reward your own, you will need to study and learn.

I do not want to mislead you about this. The book you are holding is not a book of mysticism, quackery, or magical-sounding promises. It is a book about honest and thoroughly tested medical techniques, developed by a practising psychiatrist and neurologist. I will not promise you something for nothing. Before the book ends, I will ask you to do a certain amount of studying and practising. If you are willing to do that, then the double reward can be yours.

If you are sceptical at this point, I am not greatly

concerned. I was profoundly sceptical myself when I first began to consider the use of acupuncture-related techniques in relieving pain. Most of my patients have also been sceptical when I first proposed introducing them to such treatments. But rarely has this scepticism lasted long. I am confident that yours will not last either.

One highly sceptical patient was a man in his seventies. I vividly recall how painfully he shuffled into my office, leaning on a cane, his body bent forward and twisted to one side. He was polite enough to keep his doubts to himself, but after talking with him for a few minutes, I knew perfectly well what he was thinking. His attitude was as plain as the ache in his back: he did not need to say anything about either. He was thinking, Well, I'll try anything . . . but I know it won't work.

I could not blame him for his pessimism. He had been referred to me by a houseman, who had given up on him. The houseman was the end of a long chain of practitioners who had similarly given up.

The man's ailment, stated as simply as possible, was a nerve irritation caused by a problem in one of his vertebrae or spinal bones. The problem was considered inoperable because of certain bad risks that were involved. Thus, the man had gone miserably from one practitioner to another, sometimes on referral, sometimes on his own, sometimes as a result of suggestions from friends. When he found no help in the realm of traditional medicine, he went outside it and sought other kinds of help. He visited several chiropractors without getting relief. He started a course of supposedly therapeutic yoga exercises, which made his condition much worse and landed him in bed for weeks. When all these approaches failed, he came back to traditional medicine. When I saw him, he was managing to function by gulping enormous daily quantities of aspirin and prescription medicines.

I told him that I proposed to try acupuncture. He nodded gloomily, obviously not expecting any noteworthy results.

The results, as it turned out, were much more dramatic than I had dared hope. Shortly after I inserted needles in the correct locations, the man stared at me in apparent disbelief. 'The pain went away!' he said, in a startled voice. 'It just went away!'

When he left my office, he was walking erect. There was only the slightest hint of stiffness in his gait. And he was holding his cane up in the air with both hands.

He told me later that he framed the cane and hung it on a wall of his home as a reminder. In succeeding visits, I taught him what I propose to teach you: how to administer acupuncture-like treatments to yourself, without needles, at any time of day or night and in any situation when a need arises.

Not only did my patient hang up his cane, but he abandoned his pain medications. On my advice, he continued taking anti-inflammatory drugs for a while but eventually was able to do without those as well. On his sixth and last visit to me he shook my hand with unusual warmth.

'You don't know what it's like to have my life back!' he said. 'To be able to walk, stand, sit without pain . . . You just don't know!'

As a matter of fact, I did know. There was a time in my life when I, too, was unable to walk, stand, or sit without pain in my back. But I did not tell him that. I just smiled at him and told him I was glad his backaches and his scepticism about auto-acupressure were both successfully treated.

I treated another case of scepticism involving a woman in her late thirties. I will call her Alice R. The primary sceptic in this case was not Alice R., but her surgeon.

She had consulted him because of a severe and aggravated case of herniated disc. This painful condition is often but inaccurately called 'slipped disc'. We need not go into the medical details here, except to say that the condition involves injury to one of the tough, normally flexible discs that separate the bones of the spinal column.

In many cases, given care and patience, a herniated disc will repair itself to the limited extent that the patient can live a more or less normal life by observing certain precautions. But in more severe cases, surgery is often advised. One surgical approach involves fusing together the bones on either side of the damaged disc, so that there is no longer any possibility of motion in the injured area – and, perhaps, no longer any pain.

Alice R.'s orthopaedic specialist wanted her to have this operation. However, he made no attempt to force her or trick her into it. He told her honestly what the trade-offs were. He explained that such an operation unavoidably leaves the spine less flexible than it used to be. Added demands are put on the discs on either side of the fused area. The patient must learn whole new ways of standing, walking, sitting, and lifting.

On the other hand, Alice's surgeon told her, to decline the operation might lead her to much worse trouble. Her damaged disc might repair itself. But, in his judgment, the healing process would take a long, long time. During that time, she could expect to be in serious pain on many days, perhaps most days. The only way to stand the pain, he said, would be to take large and perhaps dangerous doses of drugs.

He told her frankly that he hated to see anybody embark on a programme of long-term pill popping. She might easily become dependent on the drugs, even addicted for life. But aside from that possibility, the surgeon was worried about the hazardous side effects of large drug doses.

Balancing all these factors against each other, the doctor felt Alice's best bet would be to undergo the spinal fusion surgery. He admitted it was not an ideal solution to the problem. In his opinion, however, it involved lesser risks than the other course.

One of Alice's woman friends had recently consulted me because of chronic, disabling migraine headaches, and I had shown her how to relieve the pain with auto-acupressure. The friend had asked me many questions about the technique, and in the course of one of our talks, I had mentioned that auto-acupressure can also be used against backache. The friend passed this on to Alice, and Alice now asked her surgeon what he thought about it.

Not unnaturally, he was sceptical. He knew Alice's pain was more than trivial. It was severe enough to require more than moderate doses of powerful prescription pain-deadeners, as well as muscle relaxants. He did not see how any acupuncture-related treatment could prevail against that much pain.

'But I asked him to give me time to try it, anyway,' Alice told me as she sat in my office. She sat awkwardly and uncomfortably, her body tipped to one side in a typical backache sufferer's position. 'I just want to exhaust all the possibilities before I get on that operating table. My doctor finally said all right.' She smiled. 'He doubts this treatment will do me any good, but at least, he says, it probably can't do me any harm either.'

I nodded. 'That is certainly true. That is one of the most important differences between drugs and auto-acupressure. With auto-acupressure, it is impossible to overdose yourself.'

As it turned out, she needed only the very lightest of doses. I gave her one acupuncture treatment, using needles in the traditional way. This relieved her pain almost entirely. On a second visit, I taught her how to administer virtually the same treatment to herself, using her thumbnails instead of needles.

And then she went away. I never saw her again. But she wrote a few weeks later to give me a delighted progress report. Her backache seemed to be entirely under control without analgesic or muscle-relaxant drugs of any kind.

Moreover, her surgery had been called off. I had urged her to visit her orthopaedic specialist for regular examinations to make sure that no new damage was occurring in her back. The specialist had already told her this. In the meantime, on the basis of his latest examination, he no longer saw a reason for an immediate operation and felt fairly confident that Alice would never need one at all.

'He says he's sorry he was so sceptical,' Alice told me.

But I was in no position to blame him for his doubts. My scepticism, before I began my studies of acupuncture, was every bit as strong as his.

Chapter 3
WHY AUTO-ACUPRESSURE RELIEVES BACKACHE

A review of recent scientific journals reveals that there are several mechanisms by which acupuncture techniques may produce the relief of pain. Studies commissioned by the United States National Institutes of Health showed that acupuncture points do exist as small areas where the electric charge on the skin is altered. Stimulation of these points can produce physiological changes.

One study of stimulating acupuncture points with needles and electric current has shown that a certain type of experimentally induced pain was relieved by electro-acupuncture. The relief was equal in effectiveness to a sizable dose of intramuscular narcotic analgesic, such as 10 mg. of morphine sulphate.

The effects of acupuncture in the EEG (electro-encephalogram) were found to differ from those associated with hypnosis. In testing the efficacy of acupuncture in relieving experimental pain, *poor* hypnotic responders had as good relief as did *good* hypnotic responders. Therefore, scientists have concluded that hypnosis and acupuncture are separate and distinct methods of treatment. What the scientists produced with acupuncture, we can attempt to duplicate with auto-acupressure.

The beginnings of acupuncture are obscure. There are many legends. One often told story, for which there is no supporting evidence whatever, is that the idea of curing illnesses by needling was developed thousands of years ago in some Oriental war. Soldiers who had been superficially wounded by arrows, so the story goes, noticed that certain long-standing ills and aches were magically alleviated. From there, it was a short intellectual jump to the idea of piercing the skin less painfully and more systematically with needles.

Most such legends are probably fairy tales. Nobody even knows how old a science acupuncture is. What is known to be true is that acupuncture, whatever its roots might be, springs from social, philosophical, and scientific traditions that are quite unlike those we know in the West.

Western medicine has long been oriented toward surgery and drugs. If something goes wrong in the body, we attack it head-on. In a drastic situation, we might remove the affected part surgically. If it seems repairable, we try to repair it. However, we have a third choice. We can treat the ailment and the attendant pain and other discomfort with drugs. This all seems to make perfect sense. It seems so logical that some consider other approaches unthinkable.

In China and other parts of the East, traditional medicine avoided direct confrontation. In part, this was because social and religious customs in many regions forbade the use of corpses for learning, experimentation, and teaching. In the West, however, scientists were learning by direct observation what a heart looks like and were learning to think of it much as one might think of a mechanical pump. In the Orient, doctors had to content themselves with learning what they could by observing phenomena on the outside of the body. An entire sub-specialty of Chinese medicine, for instance, is based on subtle differences in the patient's wrist pulse. It is evaluated, not just by the rate, but by the strength, the 'depth', and other qualities that the practitioner feels with his fingertips. Having made a judgment about the 'feel' of the pulse, he translates this into a judgment about the health of the heart and other internal organs. He learns all this without actually seeing a heart or examining one physically.

Ancient practitioners of Oriental medicine were not only discouraged from examining corpses. There were also severe restrictions governing what they could and could not do to the living patient. Women often would not undress for examination or treatment, nor would men of certain social classes. Furthermore, practitioners in some communities were forbidden to spill any of the patient's blood. Sometimes, local customs or religious laws carried no restrictions against minor surgery, such as lancing a boil. However, there always were strong traditions that discouraged any major invasion of the patient's body, such as surgery inside the chest.

Thus, one main thrust of traditional Eastern medicine was toward forms of treatment that involved manipulating areas on the outside of the body. Acupuncture is only one of many such methods. Another method that achieved wide popularity in China, for instance, is moxibustion. This is a system in which various ailments are treated by heating certain carefully chosen points on the body. Those points correspond with the points chosen by acupuncturists for insertion of needles.

To the Western mind, such treatment methods seem unnecessarily indirect. This is especially accentuated when the point designated for the acupuncturist's needle (or auto-acupressurist's thumbnail) is on a body area far removed from the site of the ailment. As you will learn later in this book, many of the points designated for relief of backache and spasm are not on the back. Similarly, we have previously presented some points used to relieve headache that are nowhere near the head.

These puzzling qualities of acupuncture and related treatment systems, that is, the apparent lack of connection between the ailment and the treatment, have contributed heavily to the scepticism that has greeted such treatments in America and Europe. The sceptics' most often asked question is, 'If acupuncture works, *how* does it work?'

That is indeed a hard question to deal with. How can I relieve my backache by manipulating various body points with my thumbnails? Precisely what bodily mechanisms act to make the pain go away?

I should begin by saying that the same question is just as hard to answer when applied to aspirin or morphine. Nobody knows all about how these or other pain-deadening drugs work. It is known that they do *some things* to the nervous system and so bring about changes in the perception of pain. But what those *things* are and just how the perception of pain is made to change are still complete mysteries.

Indeed, nobody is really quite sure what pain is. The study of pain is called dolorology. It is a relatively new medical specialty in Western universities, laboratories, and hospitals. It is new mainly because the subject is so subtle and elusive. Until recently, medical scientists have despaired of making any sense out of it. Often in the past, they tried to explain themselves by proclaiming just the opposite: that the subject is *not* subtle and elusive. 'Everybody knows what pain is,' they said, 'so why study it?'

Trying to support the contention that pain is a simple matter, some scientists advanced the view that there are two kinds of pain, 'fast' and 'slow'. If you accidentally touch a hot frying pan, 'fast' pain makes you snatch your fingers away rapidly. An appreciable time later, that first sharp pain is followed by a wave of duller, less intense, 'slow' pain. Research seemed to establish that the two kinds of pain are carried by two distinct kinds of nerve fibres running directly from the site of the injury to the brain. It all seemed satisfyingly simple and tidy.

But other students of the subject began to object that there must be more varieties of pain than two. For instance, there is a distinct difference in quality between an 'aching' pain and the pain from a cut or stab. Almost everybody recognizes such differences. You can even feel both kinds simultaneously, yet separate them without any difficulty. If your back is aching at any given hour, for example, and if during that hour you happen to walk backward into a sharp-cornered piece of furniture, you can feel the old ache and the new stab at the same time, in the same body area. Such distinctions led researchers to propose more complicated schema of pain categories. In some schema there were four types of pain; in others, there were eight, and so on.

But the subject turned out to be much more complex than that. There are many kinds of bodily sensations that are perceived by some people as painful but by others as something else. Certain types of insect bites, for example, feel like 'pain' to one person but 'itch' to another. As every dentist knows, some people find that a a dental drill always produces pain. Others often describe the sensation as 'unpleasant but not actually painful'.

To make the topic still more complicated, the same person can react to the same stimulus in different ways. The reaction to pain is in part determined by what else is going on. Every athletic coach is aware of this phenomenon. Football players can get badly cut or bruised during a game. They can even break a finger or lose a tooth without seeming to feel any pain. They go on playing. The pain arrives to surprise them when the game is over.

A doctor who served the New York Jets once reported on a conversation he had with an injured man. The man had twisted his elbow joint so badly that he was unable to play for weeks afterwards. However, he completed the game in which the injury occurred. 'It was strange,' he admitted to the doctor. 'I knew I'd hurt my elbow. I mean, the message got to my brain. It said, Yeah, that elbow is in trouble. But I didn't feel the message as *pain*. The message seemed to say, Don't worry about it till later.'

Should that message be classified as a type of pain, or not?

Similarly, a US Army doctor noticed a puzzling phenomenon after a major battle in the Pacific during World War II. The doctor was in charge of a field hospital. Men were brought in with such serious wounds that in many cases, they might have been expected to be groaning in pain. Yet, as the doctor reported later, not all of them appeared to be feeling pain sensations. They conversed cheerfully. Some even seemed to be in a state of euphoria.

Why? Because they had come through the battle alive. Their wounds were tickets that would take them safely home. As one explained with a grin, 'Sure, my leg hurts. But I don't hurt.'

What message was he receiving from his leg? Should it be called pain, or something else?

Pain is obviously a much more complicated phenomenon than Western students were once taught. What makes it more puzzling still is that pain is often felt at body locations far removed from where one would expect it.

Many backache sufferers are keenly aware of this. Back problems often lead to a condition loosely referred to as sciatica, or irritation of the sciatic nerve. This may cause the sufferer to feel spears of pain shooting down one leg, sometimes all the way down to the foot. Similarly, people suffering from a heart condition called angina pectoris, which literally translated means 'chest pain', often feel pain in the left shoulder or down the left arm, far from the main locus of the problem.

I have studied acupuncture from the viewpoint of modern Western neurology and neurophysiology. My research leads me to think that the effects work somehow through the peripheral, autonomic, and central nervous systems. This is a widely accepted view, for there are many points of agreement between acupuncture and modern neurology. Many acupuncture loci, the points where needles are inserted, are located along nerve pathways with which any Western neurologist is familiar.

What has not been totally elucidated, either by the Chinese or by Westerners, is the exact neural mechanism that produces acupuncture's pain-relieving effects. Some theories state that the nervous system incorporates components called 'gates'. They operate much like a switch, controlling the passage of pain impulses from the injured site to the brain. When the gates are closed, as in those injured soldiers or football players, little or no perception of pain reaches conscious awareness. Some scientists have suggested that acupuncture works by closing such gates along various nerve pathways.

Another theory deals with a newly-discovered group of body chemicals called endorphins. These are peptides that are produced naturally in the brain and that appear to have powerful opiate-like effect. Some investigators have offered evidence that acupuncture stimulates the brain to release Beta-endorphins, which circulate throughout the body and block or impede pain messages.

The endorphin and gate-control theories are only the latest of many attempts to reconcile acupuncture with Western science. Medical researchers in Europe and America have been studying it since the seventeenth century, when it was first introduced in the West by French Jesuits returning from the Orient. A Dutch doctor, Dr William Ten Rhyne, wrote what is believed to be the first Western medical report on the subject in 1683. Like many other doctors since his time, Ten Rhyne was amazed at some of the effects he had witnessed but confessed that he was at a loss to explain them adequately.

Ten Rhyne concluded that acupuncture must be accepted on an empirical basis. That is, we can observe the effects, and we can produce the same effects again and again, reliably and repeatedly, and so we must trust those effects even though we are not certain about the cause.

Acupuncture undeniably works. Only recently have Western scientists discerned some of the mechanisms that explain *why* or *how* it works. That is undoubtedly a reason why a great deal of controversy has arisen over it. Nor is there agreement on the kinds of ailments against which it is effective. But if I confine my observations to its effectiveness in relieving certain kinds of pain and muscle spasm, I can make the statement unequivocally: *it works.* I know it does because I have seen it work on hundreds of patients and felt it work on myself. American scientists have verified the relief of experimentally induced pain by acupuncture. How useful is it? By utilizing auto-acupressure, you and your back will soon find out for yourselves.

Chapter 4
THE STRUCTURE OF THE BACK

Our spines are built of roughly ring-shaped pieces of bone called vertebrae. They rest one on top of another, very much like a tall pile of automobile tyres. Each vertebra has a hole in the centre (the vertebral foramen), through which the spinal cord passes. There are other openings in the walls of the vertebrae to admit nerves connecting the spinal cord with various parts of the body. Each vertebra has a rearward-projecting knob called a spinous process, to which muscles are attached. Other knobs and projections serve as attachments for the ribs, for ligaments, and for other purposes.

The analogy to a pile of automobile tyres is somewhat misleading, mainly for two reasons. In the first place, the vertebrae are not of equal sizes. The smallest are at the top, in the neck region. They grow progressively larger toward the bottom. In the second place, the spine is not straight. It has three major curves: forward at the neck, rearward in the region of the ribs, forward again in the lower back. A pile of tyres might be able to stand with three such curves in it, but it would not be very stable. The spine is stable because of the way in which everything is held together.

There are special names for the various parts of the spine. They are:

Cervical: the neck region, consisting of the seven smallest vertebrae. The topmost of these, and the smallest of all, supports the skull.

Thoracic: the mid-back region, consisting of twelve larger bones. These are the vertebrae to which the ribs are attached. Most people have twelve pairs of ribs. Ten of the pairs curve around to attach to the sternum or breastbone in front, while the two lower pairs are too short to meet in front and so are called 'floating' ribs. This arrangement of twelve rib pairs is not the only possible one. Some people have eleven pairs; others, thirteen.

Lumbar: the lower back, consisting of five massive vertebrae. This is the back segment that bears most of the stress in supporting the upper body. Statistically, it is the most likely to suffer breakdowns and cause pain.

The Sacrum: a large bone, shaped something like an arrowhead, that serves to anchor the lower spine to the hips. In a newborn baby, the sacrum consists of five separate vertebrae. They fuse into one massive load-bearing bone in the first years of life. This is the bone that forms the hard rear wall of your pelvic area; you can feel it just above the sharp knob of your tailbone. The part of the hipbone to which the sacrum joins on either side is called the ilium. The joint, hence, is called the sacroiliac—and it is a joint that often gives trouble.

The Coccyx (pronounced cox-ix): the tailbone. It consists of four (sometimes three) small vertebrae that usually fuse into one by adulthood. This is one part of the back that rarely gives trouble unless it is injured by a fall or blow. It sometimes becomes painful when ligaments are stretched in childbirth. The coccyx bears no weight. It may be the vestigial remainder of a tail.

These, then, are the bones of the spine: in an adult, twenty-four vertebrae plus the sacrum and coccyx. Now let us see how these twenty-six bones are held together so as to allow us to walk erect.

THE MECHANICS OF THE SPINE

The spine is a compromise between two opposing necessities. One is stability, and the other is flexibility.

Stability: The tall column of bone must be cohesive enough to maintain its essential shape while bearing a heavy weight. It must also withstand both vertical and horizontal stresses. If these twenty-six bones were hinged together as loosely as our elbows, so that each pair of vertebrae could flop back and forth over a 90-degree angle, we would never be able even to rise to a sitting posture. We would certainly be unable to stand up and walk.

Flexibility: The requirement of stability could be met by making the spine a single rigid piece of bone. But that, too, would either make most of our familiar movements impossible or would grossly curtail them. Flexibility is the second necessity. The spinal column must hold its shape—yet at the same time must be capable of bending and twisting.

The way in which nature has fulfilled these conflicting requirements is a masterpiece of engineering. In between each pair of vertebrae is a remarkable structure called an *intervertebral disc*. The disc is made mainly of extremely tough layers of ligament and cartilaginous material. But its central core consists of a softer and somewhat more flexible material called the *nucleus pulposus*.

The intervertebral discs serve several purposes. First, they help hold the spinal bones in proper alignment, one on top of another. (There are also vertical bands of ligament that further stiffen the column and preserve its shape.) Second, the discs act as cushions and separators. They absorb weight and shock. They prevent the spinal bones from grinding against each other. Third, the discs act as limiting hinges. Each disc allows a strictly limited amount of movement between the two bones that it separates. But since there are twenty-six bones, and since each is capable of moving a little in relation to its neighbours, the total amount of possible movement is large.

The spinal column rests on the pelvic girdle at the sacroiliac joint. It is held erect by thick bands of muscle in the back, belly, and buttocks.

Chapter 5
COMMON PHYSICAL CAUSES OF BACKACHE

Humans are among the longest-lived creatures on earth. During those decades of life, our spines absorb an enormous amount of punishment as we stand, walk, sit, stoop, or lift. At some time in our lives, almost *all* of us will experience pain in the back. It is certainly no cause for surprise that this structure of bones, ligaments, and other tissues is subject to a wide variety of disorders.

This chapter contains a simplified but detailed overview of the common physical causes of our backaches. It is not intended as a complete medical text or as a guide to self-diagnosis. You may wish to study this chapter in its entirety. Alternatively, you may use this chapter as an abbreviated medical encyclopaedia and review only those topics that are directly related to your specific medical problems. If you wish to do so, you will find an alphabetical index at the end of this chapter.

If your pain is chronic or regularly recurrent pain, you should consult a doctor. The causes of your pain should be diagnosed. You should then find this chapter useful as a general orientation. When you begin treating yourself with auto-acupressure, I want you to know precisely what you are treating and why.

SIMPLE TRAUMA

This term refers to the most common of all kinds of back disorders. The word *trauma* is a medical term meaning *injury* or *damage*. It does not necessarily mean a visibly serious injury. So it is with the various kinds of simple or mild trauma that can happen to the back. Obviously *something* is wrong, for pain is present. But the most careful examination, including X-ray photographs, may reveal nothing out of the ordinary. Nothing is torn or broken; nothing is out of place. The damage reveals itself only to the person feeling the pain.

There are two kinds of trauma:

Acute: The pain comes on suddenly, resulting from a fall, a blow, an abrupt and awkward lifting motion, a day spent moving furniture, a day spent in a cramped sitting position in a car. The pain is a signal that a ligament, disc, or muscle in the back has been stretched, twisted, compressed, or otherwise forced beyond its normal range of motions. Acute trauma is only one way to describe the condition. It can be called a strain, a sprain, a wrench, or any of many other terms. As long as it is a simple trauma, with no other complicating factors present, the condition can usually be handled easily enough by a few days or weeks of rest or curtailed activity, plus medication (or auto-acupressure) as needed for pain and muscle spasm.

Chronic: This refers to the kind of hidden damage that can happen to spinal structures slowly over a long span of time. The damage may result from poor standing or sitting posture, from lack of exercise leading to a weakening of abdominal and other muscles that hold the spine erect, and so on. The onset of the pain may be very slow, perhaps starting as a mild 'nagging backache' that comes and goes over a span of years, gradually growing worse. This condition, too, may turn out to be easily handled. The indicated treatment might consist of exercises to strengthen sagging muscles, better attention to posture, and auto-acupressure to control occasional bouts of pain.

MUSCLE SPASM

This is a condition that can accompany almost any injury to the back (or, for that matter, an injury anywhere in the body). In effect, it is the body's attempt to protect the injured area by preventing movement there. The muscles around the area become rigid, sometimes to such a degree that they act virtually like a hard plaster cast or a metal brace or splint. Indeed, *splinting* is one medical term used to describe the process.

Muscle spasm is undoubtedly useful during the period immediately after an injury. But what often happens is that the uncontrolled muscle contraction continues long after its usefulness has ceased. For example, muscle spasm may last long after the patient is safely installed in his bed. Then it makes sense to try to stop the spasm. Muscle spasm almost always causes pain of its own, in addition to the pain caused by the original injury.

Not only does the spasm cause pain, but it can sometimes cause damage if it continues long enough. For example, let us say you have a chronic backache caused by the effects of bad posture on the sacroiliac joint. In an attempt to take some load off the traumatized part of the joint, certain groups of muscles might become chronically tense. This pulls the spine into an awkward shape. This chronic tension could be completely unconscious on your part. You do not realize it, but you have begun to carry your body tilted to one side, or tilted backward. In time, the rigid muscles can make permanent changes in the shape of the spine, causing scoliosis, for instance (lateral or sideways curvature), or exaggerations of some of the natural curves.

There are many drugs for relieving muscle spasm, as well as for relieving pain. But as I will show you later, auto-acupressure may accomplish both purposes with considerably less danger from unwanted side effects.

DISC DAMAGE

We are now crossing the borderline from simple or mild trauma to some more complicated and serious kinds of injury. As we have seen, an intervertebral disc may be slightly compressed or twisted. It will usually repair itself without causing its owner severe or lasting pain. But if the damage is more serious—particularly if it is serious enough to be visible to an examining doctor—then the prognosis cannot be so casual.

Among the serious kinds of disc damage is a tear in the outer ligament. Still more serious is a tear and accompanying pressure of such violence that part of the nucleus pulposus is forced out through the rent. This is the painful condition called herniated or ruptured disc.

As I remarked in an earlier chapter, the layman's term is *slipped disc*—but it is a misleading term because it conjures up an altogether wrong image of what the injury actually is. There is, in fact, a spinal disorder called *spondylolisthesis*, in which a vertebra actually appears to have slipped out of its proper position. The condition is not uncommon and may cause no trouble. It oftens turns up by surprise in routine physical examinations of children and teenagers. It may cause problems in middle or old age. However, it has nothing to do with the more common kind of trauma so often called slipped disc. To avoid confusion, I will use the term 'herniated disc' from now on.

This kind of disc damage may result from some sudden, violent episode such as a fall or automobile accident. Or it may occur as a result of trying to lift a heavy object, or twisting the body while painting a ceiling. In many cases, a contributing factor may be the chronic trauma we studied before, plus the normal processes of ageing. All the body's tissues, including those in the intervertebral discs, grow progressively less elastic after young adulthood. A disc that could take a great deal of abuse when the person is twenty years old may tear or herniate under much less abuse when the person is fifty.

A disc injured in this way can repair itself with proper care. However, once your spine has undergone this kind of damage, you must treat it with new respect for the rest of your life. This does not mean that you must drastically curtail all your physical activities. It does mean that you will need to observe certain precautions (which I will outline later) and that you will probably need to start a course of special exercises to maintain the strength of muscle structures supporting your spine.

In extreme cases, a disc may be so badly torn that there is little or no hope of its repairing itself. A doctor may then determine that surgery is the only solution. There are many surgical approaches, including that of removing the destroyed disc and fusing the two neighbouring vertebrae together.

RHEUMATISM AND ARTHRITIS

These two words are used, often interchangeably, to describe a bewildering variety of diseases affecting the joints. The words *rheumatism* or *rheumatic disease* usually refer to a systemic (whole-body) disease that may affect the joints or their surrounding tissues. *Arthritis* is a general term used to describe any inflammatory condition affecting a specific joint or group of joints. (Gout is sometimes classified as a kind of arthritis.) However, the distinctions are often vague, and there is no need for us to concern ourselves with the fine points here.

What does concern us is the fact that this large group of diseases can cause, among other problems, back pain. Among the more common diseases in the group are:

Rheumatoid Arthritis: a generalized disease of the body. It attacks women more often than men and is seen most often in people aged twenty to thirty-five, but it can also affect children. The vast majority of people who contract this disease get over it with no serious long-term effects. However, about one person in ten is lastingly afflicted. The disease may start suddenly with a high fever or more slowly with a period of lassitude, aches and pains, loss of appetite. In the more serious cases, it causes irreversible and progressive damage to joint linings, so that the sufferer finds it more and more painful to move the affected joints. In extreme cases, a joint may fuse into a solid mass in which no movement is possible at all.

Ankylosing Spondylitis (also called rheumatoid spondylitis and Marie-Strümpell's disease): a disease that specifically affects the spine. It is more common in men than women, and it most often begins to manifest itself between the ages of twenty and thirty. The earliest symptom is often a nagging ache in the lumbar region, slowly worsening with time. The ache is caused by abnormal hardening or loss of elasticity in ligaments and other spinal tissues. In many patients, for reasons that are not understood, the progression of the disease stops spontaneously before the trouble is serious. But in others, it may progress until parts of the spine are virtually immobilized. In extreme cases, the entire spine grows rigid from the neck to the sacroiliac—so rigid that the ribs cannot move, and the patient has trouble breathing.

The following five factors are typical discriminators of ankylosing spondylitis: (1) onset of back discomfort before the age of forty years, (2) insidious onset of pain, (3) persistence for more than three months, (4) association with morning stiffness, and (5) improvement with exercise.

Osteoarthritis (also called degenerative or 'wear-and-tear' arthritis): a condition that most often appears in middle or old age. It is characterized by a general wearing away of the cartilaginous tissues that form the bearing surfaces of joints, notably in the spine. Nearly everybody exhibits such joint changes by age fifty or sixty. But in the majority of men and women the changes cause only mild occasional pain and stiffness. In some, however, the changes progress fast enough to cause more serious pain and sometimes crippling stiffness. What happens is that cartilage lining the joints can disintegrate entirely, leaving bone grinding against bone.

Psoriatic Arthritis: the name given to certain arthritic changes that often accompany the skin disease, psoriasis. The skin disease itself is not well understood, but is believed to stem from a possibly inherited error in metabolism. It can be controlled and its symptoms alleviated, but no complete cure has yet been discovered. For reasons that remain largely mysterious, people afflicted with psoriasis have a high incidence of rheumatoid arthritis and other joint diseases.

CONGENITAL DEFECTS

Surprisingly large numbers of people—about half the population, according to one widely accepted estimate—have congenital defects of the spine and its associated structures. In most cases, however, to call them 'defects' is something of an exaggeration. They may be nothing more than trivial deviations from the norm. They may cause little or no trouble, and may not be discovered until late in life. The person with such a defect may live a full, long and active life, without becoming aware of any back problem. However, such defects do, in many cases, cause or contribute to occasional or frequent back pains.

Spina bifida, to take one example, is a condition in which the base of the spine fails to fuse properly—almost as though a piece of bone has been left out. In its severe form, this malformation can cause lifelong total paralysis of the lower body and perhaps early death. However, in a less severe form—called spina bifida occulta, meaning 'hidden'—it may be the cause of nothing much more than the inconvenience of a mild and infrequent backache.

I have already mentioned another such congenital defect, spondylolisthesis, the condition in which a vertebral body is imperfectly aligned with its neighbours. This, too, may go unnoticed until late in life. Then it may begin to cause pain as the surrounding structures succumb to the normal weakening and loss of elasticity that accompany old age.

Another relatively common defect is an abnormal connection or fusion of the sacrum and the fifth (lowest) lumbar vertebra. Depending on the way in which it occurs, this is called either lumbarization of the sacrum or sacralization of the lumbar vertebra. It leads to a certain loss of suppleness in the lower back, but the person with the defect may not experience this as a problem. The stiffness in that area may be wholly or partly compensated for by more than normal flexibility in other parts of the spine. However, the defect may cause backache under various circumstances, particularly in middle or old age.

DISORDERS OF SPINAL CURVATURE

Scoliosis is an appreciable sideways (or lateral) curvature in the normally straight vertical line of the spine. The deformity may be no more than a temporary disturbance produced by the spinal muscles. Or it may be structural with permanent changes in the bones or soft tissues.

Idiopathic scoliosis is the most important type of structural scoliosis. It is called idiopathic because its cause is unknown. It accounts for 80 to 90 per cent of scoliosis cases. It begins in childhood or adolescence and tends to increase progressively until skeletal growth stops.

Lumbar scoliosis may occur to counteract the effect of a sideways tilt in the pelvis. This tilt may occur because the lower limbs are unequal in length or because of deformity at the hip joint.

Sciatic scoliosis is the term sometimes used to describe the deformity resulting from muscle spasm, which we looked at earlier. In sciatic scoliosis, the lumbar part of the spine may list away from the affected side.

Kyphosis is the medical term for an excessive backward curvature of the spinal column. In hunchback, there is an abnormally increased curvature of the thoracic spine as viewed from the side. In the cervical and lumbar regions, where there is normally a forward curvature, any reversal of this constitutes cervical or lumbar kyphosis.

Lordosis is the forward curvature of the spinal column. Normal lordosis is the usual forward curvature in the neck and lumbar regions. However, lordosis is also commonly used to refer to abnormally increased frontward curvature of the spinal column. Abnormal lordosis is the opposite deformity to kyphosis.

A flat back is one that has a decrease in the normal lumbar lordosis and normal thoracic kyphosis. In hollowback, saddleback, and swayback, there is an exaggerated lordosis of the lumbar spine. In many cases, abnormal lumbar lordosis is caused by poor posture. The condition may also be associated with enlargement of the abdomen, such as may occur with obesity and pregnancy.

TUMOURS

There are many, many kinds of tumours or growths that can afflict the spine and its surrounding tissues. They can grow on the bone, in the spinal canal, on nerve tissues, on muscles, on connecting tissues. All of them can cause pain.

Some tumours are benign—meaning that they do not display wild uncontrolled growth and do not threaten to metastasize or 'seed' themselves in other parts of the body. A fairly common type of benign tumour is a meningeoma. It is a growth on the tissue around the brain and spinal cord. Another type is a tumour that grows around a nerve root emerging from an opening in a vertebra. Such a tumour is called a neurinoma or schwannoma.

Though benign, such tumours can cause a great deal of trouble and may need to be removed surgically, for example, a tumour that grows inside the spinal canal where the space is rigidly limited. The result could be pressure on nerves or damage to the nerves and their protective tissues. The amount of space inside the spinal canal varies greatly from one person to another. This may become a factor in determining whether a benign tumour is troublesome. In some people, a relatively small tumour can be hazardous. In others with more space in the canal, a larger benign tumour might produce few symptoms or none. In such a case, the doctor might decide that surgery would involve greater risk for the patient than simply leaving the tumour alone.

A malignant or cancerous tumour, by contrast, cannot be treated so casually. Such a tumour grows wildly, invades surrounding tissues, and has the frightening property of spreading to distant body sites through the bloodstream or lymphatic system.

Primary spinal bone tumours—that is, cancers which get their start in the vertebral bones—are fortunately not common. But there are many types of cancer that are known to attack the spine, particularly in older people. Among the most feared is multiple myeloma, a tumour of the bone marrow.

More common are the so-called secondary tumours—those that get their start elsewhere in the body and spread to the spinal column. Because of the extremely rich blood supply around the vertebral bodies, such metastatic seeding happens more often than one would wish. Among the more common sites of origin are the breast, prostate, kidneys, lung, and thyroid. A malignant tumour in any of those sites represents a potential threat to the spine.

There are many varieties of malignancy, and they act

in many different ways. Some bone tumours will increase the density of the bone they attack, while others will decrease it. All, of course, are dangerous. This is one more excellent reason why anybody with persistent back pain should not merely treat the symptom but should consult a doctor regularly.

Unfortunately, metastatic bone tumours do not always signal their presence promptly. A single standard X-ray examination may not detect anything until as much as one-fourth to one-third of the given bone area has been replaced by tumour. Other kinds of tests can provide an earlier warning. If a doctor examines you on a regular basis, it is likely that he will observe various changes and other clues that will suggest the need for such tests.

FRACTURES AND DISLOCATIONS

Malignancies such as those we have just considered can soften or weaken a vertebra to such an extent that a trivial accident—a mere bump or awkward twisting movement—can break it. When a doctor sees a vertebral fracture and learns that it occurred so easily, malignancy is among the first possibilities that will cross his mind.

Fractures can occur in perfectly healthy bone too. The typical spinal break is the compression fracture. It results from a downward crushing force on the spinal column. In healthy bone this most often occurs as a result of violent trauma: an automobile accident, a serious fall, or an attempt to stop a heavy object from falling. At such times, enormous force can be exerted against the vertebral bodies, and one or more of them may crack. The typical compression fracture shows up on X-rays as a wedge-shaped break line, and it is sometimes accompanied by herniation of one or more neighbouring discs. It can be agonizingly painful. But as long as there are no complications such as injury to nerve roots or the spinal cord, it usually responds to proper care.

A violent fall or accident may also push a vertebra out of proper alignment instead of breaking it. This might result in a condition called *subluxated facet*, in which one of the vertebra's bony spurs is forced into a faulty position. Sometimes this condition, which is usually very painful, can be relieved by chiropractic techniques or some similar manipulation.

Another possible result of violent trauma is spondylolisthesis—which, as we have seen, can also occur as a congenital malformation. In the typical case, the vertebra slips forward in relation to the two on either side of it. The condition may correct itself in time. On the other hand, it may be severe enough to threaten damage to nerve roots or the spinal cord itself. In such a case, a doctor might advise spinal fusion or some other surgery to prevent serious after-effects.

METABOLIC DISEASES

Many of the disorders under this heading may also be classified under arthritis or rheumatism, those large, loose categories we looked at earlier.

One metabolic disease that frequently causes pain in the back (as well as other joints) is *gout*. Gout is an inherited disease. Because of an inborn error of metabolism, the body produces more uric acid than it can absorb in its normal chemical processes or pass out in urine. The result is that urates, or uric acid salts, are deposited in various parts of the body, including joints of the spine and hips. These chalky deposits, called tophi, can seriously interfere with the mechanical working of the joint, and can cause a great deal of pain and inflammation.

The disease is more common in men than women. It does not often manifest itself before age thirty. In many people, it causes virtually no trouble at all. The high uric acid content may only be discovered during a routine blood test. The urate deposits, if any, may occur in places where they are barely noticed, such as the cartilage of the ears. But in other people, gout can be a crippling disease. Fortunately, it can usually be controlled with proper medication, which is used in one form to relieve the symptoms of an acute attack and in another to prevent the formation of excessive amounts of uric acid.

Gout is probably more common than most people realize. Indeed, it is likely that many people suffer from its less severe forms without ever realizing they have it. The symptoms may be occasional aching in the back or other joints, and the sufferer may pass it off as a sprain or strain. This in itself may be all right—but problems could arise if the sufferer then takes aspirin for the pain. One of aspirin's chemical side effects is that it can elevate the concentration of uric acid in the blood. Thus, an unaware gout sufferer who swallows a lot of aspirin over a span of years might eventually develop severe symptoms. Auto-acupressure, of course, has no such side effects.

Another metabolic disease that can affect the spine is *osteomalacia*, a softening of bone resulting from disturbances in calcium metabolism. In adults, the disorder resembles rickets in children.

Osteoporosis is another such disorder, but it can develop from any of several causes. It is characterized by a loss of mineral content in the bones and a consequent softening and weakening, as the bones become increasingly porous and brittle. It can result from hormonal changes such as menopause or adrenal overactivity (Cushing's syndrome); from long-term fad dieting or other kinds of poor nutrition; or from vascular abnormalities of various kinds.

The typical osteoporosis patient is a woman in post-menopausal years who consults a doctor about low backache. Her height may have decreased quite markedly in recent years—a common symptom of this disease. X-ray examinations may reveal still another tell-tale symptom: one or more small fractures in the vertebrae. We noted before that certain tumours can weaken bone to the extent that trivial accidents will break it, and the same is true of osteoporosis. Often, indeed, a patient will not be able to recall *any* specific episode to explain a vertebral fracture. This will immediately suggest to an examining physician that something is seriously wrong with the bone. Osteoporosis will be among the first possible explanations that spring to his mind.

LOCALIZED BONE DISEASES

The diseases we looked at in the preceding section are considered general metabolic diseases. They spring from metabolic errors and omissions affecting the whole body and may produce their symptoms anywhere in the body. Gout, for instance, can affect any joint or all joints. Osteomalacia can affect any bone or all bones. In contrast to these general diseases, there are some diseases that attack bones in a localized body area only.

Prominent among these is osteitis deformans, or *Paget's disease*. It never attacks all the bones but confines itself to one or a few sites, often including the spine. The main symptom is a severe disturbance in the process of new bone formation. In healthy bone, this process goes on at a measured pace, with old bone cells dying and new cells continually replacing them. In Paget's disease, the destruction of old bone becomes much more rapid than normal. The newly-formed bone that replaces it is not properly constructed. After the disease has been present for a time, the bone takes on a peculiar moth-eaten appearance.

Paget's disease and its causes are not well understood. It is particularly baffling because its course can never be predicted with any confidence. In some patients, its progress will abruptly and mysteriously halt. In some cases, the disease may resume years later. In others, the progress is continual but very slow. These patients may have backache, but perhaps no major inconvenience until old age. But, where progress is fast, patients may experience severe pain and frequent vertebral fractures, and may be crippled at a relatively early age.

INFECTIOUS DISEASES

Some of these diseases, too, are often classified as varieties of arthritic or rheumatic afflictions. For example, we have already considered rheumatic fever. Flu, colds, and other common infectious diseases can also cause inflammation and stiffness in joints. Certain other diseases such as tuberculosis can produce bone and joint infections.

More common in the United States are pyogenic (pus-forming) infections. Such infections may be either acute (rapidly rising to a climax) or chronic. Acute pyogenic infections of the spine and surrounding tissues often arise from infections elsewhere in the body—typically from the lungs in children, the urinary tract in adults. Fortunately, most such spinal infections respond to treatment quite rapidly if caught in time. With proper care, they usually subside without doing permanent damage to bone or other tissues. However, they can cause considerable pain and inconvenience while they are still active.

Chronic infections may be harder to control. For example, one type that is quite common in the USA today is chronic pyogenic osteomyelitis, a potentially dangerous and almost always painful bone inflammation. It can get its start from an unclean wound that discharges bacteria and poisons into the bloodstream. The infection may lodge in bones far removed from the original wound. Among the sufferers being seen most frequently by doctors today are drug addicts who have habitually injected themselves with unsterilized needles.

CIRCULATORY DISORDERS

Certain disorders of the circulatory system can mimic sciatica (pain involving the sciatic nerve) and other symptoms of a herniated disc. The patient may feel pain in the lower back, perhaps spreading to one buttock and leg or both. The entire lumbar and hip region may feel stiff; walking or stooping may hurt, and so on. The patient may feel quite certain that the problem is a traumatized disc, when in fact the real cause of the pain is something much more serious.

Circulatory disorders that produce low backache are not as common as herniated discs, but they are not rare. I make this point to illustrate, once again, the hazards of self-diagnosis. If your back hurts—and particularly if the pain starts abruptly with no readily apparent reason—you should consult a doctor.

One condition that can produce this misleading kind of backache is *Leriche's syndrome*. This is a clot in the abdominal aorta, a large blood vessel that passes close to the lumbar spine. Another such condition is an *aneurysm* in that same abdominal aorta. An aneurysm is a balloon-like swelling at a point where the walls of a blood vessel have been weakened by disease, a congenital defect, or some other cause. Such a swelling in the abdominal aorta can impinge on one of the lumbar vertebrae or on nerve roots, causing a deep-boring pain.

Statistically, the most likely candidate for this kind of trouble is a man aged fifty or older with a history of arteriosclerosis, or hardening of the arteries. In the recent past, he may have been unusually troubled by cold feet and may also have had several small strokes.

INDEX TO PHYSICAL CAUSES

Chapter 6
COMMON EMOTIONAL PROBLEMS THAT CAUSE BACKACHE

Not all back pains necessarily have tangible physical causes. There are many psychological mechanisms that could make the pain seem worse. Psychological causes also could make the pain last months or years longer than can be explained by the physical damage alone. I see such cases often in my work as a psychiatrist. Among the more common:

You-owe-me backache. Insurance investigators and lawyers who handle accident-compensation cases frequently deal with this phenomenon. Very often, a backache will last until all the legal and financial questions of a compensation case are settled, and then will miraculously disappear.

This sounds more cynical than it is meant to be. True, some backaches are consciously and deliberately faked. But in many other cases, the patient actually does feel the pain. He clings to it, refusing to believe that it is subsiding, because to lose it would be to suffer a financial loss. No amount of testimony by insurance doctors or badgering by lawyers will shake his own belief in the pain. To him, it is perfectly real.

The reason for the backache need not be money. It

could be one of a large number of reasons, such as a need for love. The person with a backache may be saying to friends or family members: You must pay attention to me, and take care of me, because I am in pain. As in the compensation case, this sufferer feels pain because he or she *wants* to feel it. To lose it would be to lose all those special privileges and extra doses of affection that an invalid can command.

I-need-treatment backache. When a patient consults a doctor about backache, the real problem could lie elsewhere. The patient might have a sexual problem and might be embarrassed to talk about it. He or she might suspect the presence of some dread disease, may want it diagnosed but may be afraid to mention it.

Again, there is no need to assume the backache is faked. The sufferer may experience real pain. The pain is the body's way of presenting itself for treatment. The patient is telling the doctor, in effect: I am ill, but I want you to discover the real problem by yourself.

The excuse-me backache. A backache can be made to serve as an explanation for many kinds of failure: in sex and family relationships, in one's career, and so on. The sufferer is saying: Of course my sexual drives are weak. Yours would be too if your back hurt the way mine does. Or: You can't imagine how hard it is to concentrate on work with this kind of constant pain.

The all-purpose cop-out. Backaches, like headaches, can be used to get us out of unpleasant tasks, unwelcome social obligations, and anything else we do not want to do. For instance:

'I'm afraid you'll have to run the meeting without me. My back seems to be acting up again.'

'I was planning to invite you out to dinner, but my back . . .'

'I know you're short of volunteers and I'd really like to help, but . . .'

'I was going to spend the weekend cleaning out the cellar, but . . .'

'You know how much I wanted to do it tonight, but my back . . .'

The I-have-emotional-problems backaches. Backaches often turn up as a physical manifestation of emotional pain. A common example is in a typical mid-life crisis. A person arriving at middle age may be seized by a feeling of not having made it in life. He may feel he has not achieved his youthful goals or measured up to some external ideal of success. This very common kind of crisis often gives rise to various kinds of physical problems; they are, in effect, the body's way of expressing that emotional despondency. Frequent or chronic backaches are typical of such unhappy situations.

In many cases, there are tangible physical reasons for low backache. All are traceable to the emotional problems that are at the root of the crisis. The feelings of inadequacy and depression can lead to harmful changes in the sufferer's personal habits: lack of exercise, sagging posture, loss of appetite, excessive drinking, smoking, and so on. Such changes can undermine a man's or woman's general health and can exacerbate the kinds of chronic back trauma we studied earlier. The result: backache. Completing the circle, the pain may plunge the sufferer into still deeper emotional despair.

Excuse for drug taking. Many men and women, in the course of treatment for a back disorder, do become insidiously dependent on analgesics, muscle relaxants, or tranquillizers. Frequently, multiple drug dependency occurs. They find that they want to continue taking their drugs long after the damaged back has repaired itself and the physical cause of the pain no longer exists. To postpone the feared day when they must abandon their pills, they convince themselves that the pain is still there.

This is not just a problem of the relatively unusual patient who develops a morphine-type addiction to some powerful prescription drug. On the contrary, the problem is widespread. It is quite possible to become psychologically dependent on a mild tranquillizer, an over-the-counter analgesic, or any drug that produces alterations in bodily sensations or moods. The relaxing effects of such a drug may become inextricably woven into the fabric of daily living. The drug makes life's sharp edges less sharp. In time, the patient comes to depend on it as an aid in facing stress and coping with everyday problems. The patient tells himself and other people: 'I am taking these pills for an entirely acceptable reason. I must control the pain in my back.'

It may also happen that the patient continues taking drugs because of fear that pain will return. As many backache sufferers know only too well, herniated discs and other back disorders can be intensely agonizing. Remembering the pain and understandably fearing it, the sufferer may go on swallowing analgesics and other drugs long after the physical pain has left. This person can very easily convince himself or herself that the dreaded pain is lurking down there as before: that the pain is waiting to return at the first sign of a lapse in vigilant pill popping. 'I can feel the pain beginning to build up whenever a pill starts to wear off,' the patient insists. It is often hard for a doctor or anyone else to convince such a patient that the feared backache may only be fear. These patients are so certain the pain exists that in their minds it does.

Chapter 7
LISTENING TO DOCTORS TALK ABOUT BACKS

The previous chapters have not attempted to cover every conceivable cause of backache, but rather to give you some brief insights into the complexity of the subject. Your own backaches may have many causes, some physical, some emotional. Identifying them and sorting them out is a task for your doctor. But it is likely that you can help him in making the diagnosis and choice of treatment. Later you can be an effective participant in that treatment, if you have an informal layman's knowledge of the spine and the many problems it may encounter. That is why I believe you will find this chapter useful.

In talking about your particular case, your doctor may use different terms and phrases than I have used. It is also likely that your well-meaning friends, neighbours, and family members will attempt to make laymen's spot diagnoses of your problem. They may confuse you with still other terms, slipped disc, for instance. Back disorders are so common that it often seems as if a separate language has grown up around them. In order to understand your own problem, here is a very brief glossary of the more common terms that a backache victim is likely to hear in and out of a doctor's office:

Nonarticular Rheumatism. This is a medical term encompassing all those diseases and conditions that involve the soft tissues around joints, but do not directly involve the joints themselves. The most common types of nonarticular rheumatism are grouped under another medical term: fibrositis.

Fibrositis. This, again, is not the name of a specific condition but is a catch-all word. It refers to painful, inflammatory conditions involving ligaments, muscles, muscle tendons, and so on. The simple trauma we looked at earlier might often be classed as a variety of fibrositis. Or the inflammation and other problems might occur because of some systemic infection such as influenza or the common cold.

Lumbago. This is more a layman's term than a medical one. It means any undiagnosed pain in the lumbar region, the small of the back. There is no specific disease called 'lumbago'. At one time, medical authorities did use the word to describe what they thought was a specific condition, but that was in a day when little was known about spinal disorders such as gout or the herniated disc. Now that it is possible to name such disorders more specifically, 'lumbago' has more or less passed out of usage.

Sciatica. This is the name of a symptom, not a disease. In many back disorders, but especially in cases of disc injury, roots of the sciatic nerve get irritated. The sciatic nerve is a great bundle of nerve fibres, the longest in the body, with its roots in the lower back. (Its name means 'hip joint nerve'.) The nerve splits into two main pathways and goes through the buttock muscles and down the legs into the feet. When the roots in the lumbar region are irritated, the sufferer may feel 'referred' pain in one buttock and leg, sometimes in both. The pain may go clear down to the foot. In about 70 per cent of cases, it is accompanied by sensations of numbness or weakness in the legs, knees, or ankles. Often the sufferer finds it hard to move the straightened leg forward for more than a few inches. Unless the pain is caused by disease or injury directly involving the sciatic nerve itself, the condition usually subsides as the back injury repairs itself.

If you suffer back pains from a disorder not mentioned in this brief chapter, please refer to the appropriate section in the previous two chapters. In Chapters 5 and 6, there is a more detailed discussion of the common physical and emotional causes of backache. All the conditions listed in Chapters 5, 6, and 7 can be associated with pain and muscle spasm.

Chapter 8
THE BASIC PRINCIPLES OF RELIEVING BACKACHE WITH AUTO-ACUPRESSURE

You are now about to learn a new way of relieving back pains. Since it is new to you, you should expect an initial period of unfamiliarity and awkwardness. During this period, your results may be disappointing.

This initial period is, in effect, a period of 'apprenticeship'. It is quite brief for most people. But I want to be very sure you are prepared for it. There is almost always such a period. Auto-acupressure utilizes the application of acupuncture-like techniques to oneself. It is not a particularly difficult skill to master, but it is a skill; it must be learned. Your confidence and the sureness of your fingers and thumbs will improve with practice. So will the efficacy of the technique in relieving pain and muscle spasm.

I make a point of this because I do not want you to give in to early disappointment. This is not a book of quackery. It makes no promises that it cannot fulfil. Some of my patients have used words like 'miraculous' and 'magical' in describing auto-acupressure, and some have talked about 'instant' relief, but to promise such results would be foolhardy. Auto-acupressure depends on the proper stimulation of nerves at certain very carefully chosen body points or loci. Except by luck, you are not likely to find the loci precisely or stimulate them in the right way the first time you try.

When you become skilled with the technique, however, you will find that the relief may come faster and more surely than is possible with pills.

In the next chapters, you will find illustrated descriptions of the major locations to stimulate for relief of backache, along with specific instructions dealing with stimulation of each locus. This chapter is devoted to general directions. Be sure to familiarize yourself thoroughly with what is said here before attempting your first self-treatment.

PREPARATIONS

If you are under a doctor's care for your back problem, ask his advice before you start using auto-acupressure. This is only common sense. In designing your course of treatment, he may well have had to balance many factors against each other. To make *any* change without consulting him would be foolish and might be dangerous. It is likely that your doctor will endorse your use of auto-acupressure. However, he might want to make certain other changes in your treatment programme to accommodate this new element. Auto-acupressure should be included as part of a total medical treatment programme.

Be wary of making abrupt changes in your drug-taking regimen, especially if you are on prescription drugs. You are quite likely to find that auto-acupressure can replace analgesics and muscle relaxants. But *do not* stop taking any prescribed drug until the doctor who prescribed it has said you may. One reason for this is that abrupt withdrawal from some drugs can be physically dangerous. Another reason is that many drugs have multiple effects. While auto-acupressure can control pain and muscle spasm, it may not produce other effects that your doctor feels are needed. Your doctor may be delighted to have you reduce your daily intake of analgesics, but he may want you to take some medication to reduce inflammation.

THE THUMBNAIL TECHNIQUE

Auto-acupressure is derived from acupuncture. However, it would be very dangerous for most people to stimulate themselves with needles. Needle acupuncture should be administered only under the watchful eye of a doctor. For that reason, in treating your backache you will be using your thumbnails instead of needles.

Be sure you understand this clearly. Pressing with the fleshy pads or bony tips of your thumbs may have little or no effect on the nerves you are attempting to stimulate. You *must* use the nails.

Your thumbnails should be short and rounded so that you do not injure yourself with your own nails. To make certain you do not, I would counsel against trying this technique with long or pointed nails. Plastic nail extenders are definitely hazardous. When auto-acupressure is properly applied, there is *no* bruising, puncturing, or any other injury which can affect the skin.

Your thumbs should be *bent* when applying auto-acupressure. This is illustrated in Fig. 1.

The human hand is built in such a way that the thumb can apply maximum pressure when in this bent position. To improve the leverage still more, I will suggest various ways in which you can oppose the pressure from your thumb with answering pressure from your fingers. For example, when your bent thumb is pressing the thumbnail into a point on one side of your leg, your fingers will be wrapped around the other side.

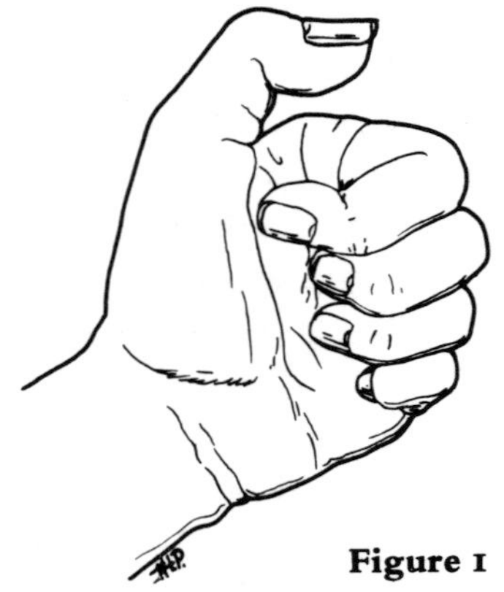

Figure 1

HOW MUCH PRESSURE?

You must press on the indicated points hard enough to make them hurt briefly. As you will discover, some of them will be exquisitely tender. (In fact, the tenderness will be a signal that you have hit the given locus with precision.) Do not worry: the pain will not last long, and your reward for enduring it will be the alleviation of much longer-lasting pain in your back. But you *must* be willing to press hard enough to affect the nerve at the indicated locus. Insufficient pressure will not produce the desired effects.

HOW LONG?

Maintain hard pressure for 30 seconds at each acupressure point.

If you find it difficult to maintain pressure steadily for that long a time, try a rhythmic on–off technique instead. In this technique, you increase and decrease the pressure once a second throughout the 30-second period. Push hard; then ease off; then push again.

CHOOSING AUTO-ACUPRESSURE POINTS

In the next chapters, you will find descriptions and illustrations of pairs of points in various parts of the back, thighs, legs, and ears. Obviously, you will not want to use all these points every time your back aches. Instead, you should choose among them on the basis of two main questions:

1. *Which are most effective for me?* An excellent way to start answering this question is to experiment. Start with those points which are the most tender when your

back is aching. They are tender because they are on nerve pathways that are being stimulated by referred pain from the site of the back disorder. These particular points are most likely to produce results when stimulated by auto-acupressure.

Having found which are the most tender points, experiment with various combinations. You should be able to find two or three pairs of points that have a clear effect on your backache. If there are no points that seem clearly more tender than the others, then it will be a process of trial and error. However, most people discover highly effective points quite rapidly.

2. *Which are the easiest for me to stimulate?* Not everybody is shaped alike. All people do not have the same dexterity and muscular strength in their hands. Not all points are equally accessible to all men and women. Furthermore, as a backache sufferer, you may well have more stiffness in the back and hips on some days than on others. A point you could reach easily yesterday may seem inaccessible today.

If you discover that several different pairs of points give you approximately equal results, choose among them on the basis of accessibility. If a point seems hard for you to reach and is awkward to stimulate, abandon the point. Work with others that are more accessible.

PAIRING

I have used the phrase *pairs of points*, and now I will explain what I mean by it. With exceptions, most acupressure points come in matched pairs: one on the left side of the body and a corresponding point on the right. For example, one backache locus is behind the left knee, and the matching one is behind the right knee.

As a general rule, you will usually find points most tender on the side of the body where the back pain is. If your back-pain is clearly one-sided, you might feel it sharply on the right side, perhaps radiating downward through the right buttock. In that case, you might find that all or most of the pressure points on your right side are much more tender than the matching ones on the left. If that is so, you may find that you can obtain adequate or complete relief simply by applying auto-acupressure to those right-side points. However, if the points on the opposite side are more sensitive than normal, the most complete pain relief may be obtained from stimulating both sides.

There may be a crossover effect. Your pain might be on one side, and the most tender acupressure points might be on the opposite side. For example, your pain is on the right side, but your most tender points are on the left side. When that is the case, it is possible that you may obtain relief just by stimulating the points on the left side. Again, it is much more likely that stimulation of acupressure points on both the right and left sides will obtain the best results.

It may also happen that your backache is not clearly located on either side. It may feel centred or diffused, with no readily apparent location at all. In this case, there is not likely to be too much difference between left and right in the tenderness of the loci. Some pairs may be more tender than other pairs, as we noted earlier; but the two points in each pair are likely to be quite evenly matched. In any situation such as this, where there is anything less than a perfectly clear difference in tenderness from left to right, you should press *both* points in each pair.

REPEAT APPLICATIONS

When you follow the directions in this book, it is impossible to 'overdose' yourself with auto-acupressure. This is not true of drugs, of course.

If you find that an initial application of auto-acupressure has not given you adequate relief (which is likely to happen frequently during your apprenticeship period, less often later), you simply repeat the process. When one application begins to 'wear off', you should be able to give yourself another with perfect safety.

If an initial application has not worked well, you may find it helpful to vary the technique or loci the second time you try. This will be especially useful in your early, experimental period. If you used steady pressure the first time, try the rhythmic off-on technique the next time. If you pressed only the points on one side and did not get sufficient pain relief, stimulate the points on both sides during the repeat application.

POSITION

All the points should be pressed while you are sitting or lying down. As we go through the points one by one, I will describe the positions that most people seem to find the most effective. You can vary these if you wish. However, do not try to apply pressure while standing.

This concludes our discussion of basic principles. You are now ready to learn how to relieve your backache with the auto-acupressure system of body points.

Chapter 9
THE BODY-POINT SYSTEM: METHODS OF LOCATION

The Auto-Acupressure System of Body Points deals with large nerves that become involved in backache. One such nerve is the sciatic, whose branches and subdivisions make it by far the longest nerve pathway in the body. The auto-acupressure points in this body system are all points where branches of such nerves come close enough to the skin surface to be accessible to thumbnail pressure.

In the pages that follow, I will describe the system of body points one by one, giving you directions to help you find each point. Follow the directions as carefully as you can, referring to the drawings for further guidance. As I mentioned in the last chapter, it is *essential* that you locate each point precisely. Even a very small deviation from the target could lessen the thumbnail pressure's effects and sometimes make the entire process ineffective. In auto-acupressure, a miss is as good as a mile. For full effect, you must learn to press exactly on the points where nerves are most fully exposed.

This will not be as difficult as it sounds. Your body will tell you when you are on target. When you learn to recognize them, the signals will be unmistakable.

To some degree, every auto-acupressure point is more sensitive to thumbnail pressure than are the surrounding areas. This is true even when your back is not aching and the nerves are not in a particularly irritated state. When you press your thumbnail firmly and precisely into one of the designated points, you will feel a peculiar sensation of tenderness. To many people, the sensation is something like the tingling that results when you hit the 'funny bone' at the back of your elbow. That odd feeling does not come from hitting bone, but from hitting a nerve that is exposed between the bones in the elbow joint. The sensation seems to spread down the outer side of your arm, sometimes into the palm of your hand and down the little finger. The sensation that results from thumbnailing an acupressure point is seldom quite so dramatic but is similar. There is a feeling of having hit a nerve, which is precisely what you have done.

At times when your back is aching, many or most of those same points will become especially tender. Thus, if you have trouble locating any point when you are not actually suffering from backache, wait until the next backache strikes. Then you are likely to find that some hard-to-find points are signalling their positions with great clarity.

MEASURING

It is essential in auto-acupressure (as in traditional acupuncture) to locate points *exactly*. If you are even as little as a quarter-inch off target, in many cases you may find that you get disappointing results.

This chapter makes use of drawings to help you find the acupressure points on your own body. I will also give written directions. In doing so, I will use certain units of measurement that may be unfamiliar to you; they may seem puzzlingly imprecise. I will be talking about *finger widths* and *finger inches*. What are they? Why do I use them instead of more familiar units?

The reason for using them is not hard to explain. Human beings do not come in one standard size. A given acupressure point might be 6 inches from the knee in somebody with long legs, but only 4 inches in somebody with short legs. Thus, any attempt to use fixed units of measurement such as inches would lead us into confusion.

Though people differ in size and shape, certain body *relationships*, however, are almost always constant. Certain dimensions of the hands, for example, tend to maintain a quite constant relationship with other body dimensions in a given person. Thus, if you use your hands to measure distances on *your* body, you are likely to arrive at the same points as somebody else using his hands to mark off distances on *his* body.

Hence my use of variable rather than fixed units of measurement. In describing them to you, I will use a few anatomical terms for the sake of precision. If you examine your hand, you will see that each finger is built of three segments, called *phalanges*, while your thumb has only two. The anatomical terms for the phalanges are:

Distal: the outer phalange—the one bearing the fingernail or thumbnail.

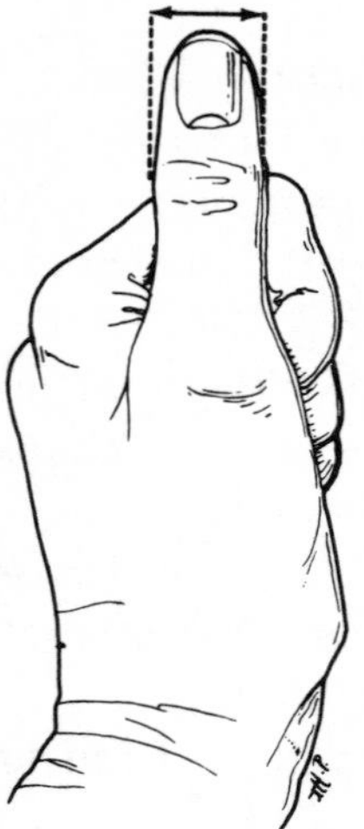

Figure 2

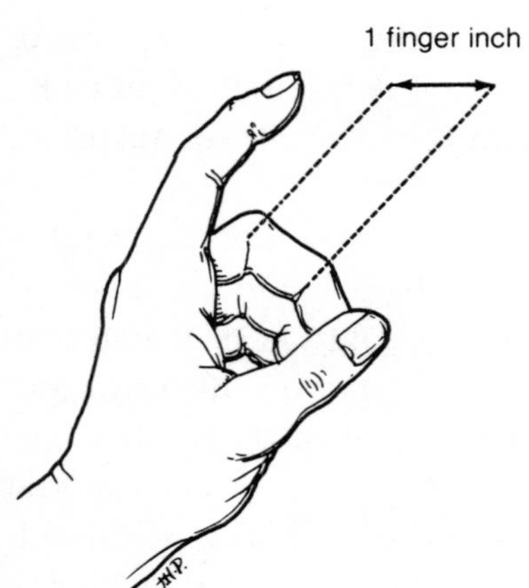

Figure 3

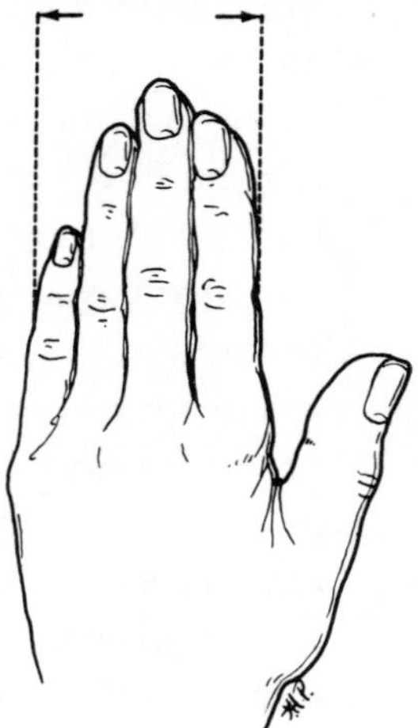

Figure 4

Middle: the next one in. The thumb has no middle phalange.

Proximal: the inner one—the finger segment on which you might wear a ring.

Now look at the drawings. They illustrate the two variable measurements commonly used in acupuncture and auto-acupressure:

Finger width: the width of one proximal phalange.

Finger inch: the width of the distal phalange of the thumb. Or—an alternative way to arrive at it—the distance between the two creases or folds in the middle of your middle finger: the creases at the two ends of the middle phalange.

Four finger widths should equal roughly three finger inches. Check this with your own hands, using both methods of finding the finger inch. With one hand stretched out flat, fingers together, use the other hand to mark off three finger inches across the four proximal phalanges. You may find that the four-to-three ratio works out more precisely with one method of measuring the finger inch than with the other. If so, abandon the less accurate method.

These variable measurements are not accurate to the last millimetre. But they will help you find the approximate locations of the pressure points. Once you are probing near a point, you will usually be able to locate it quickly by being alert to the special sensation of tenderness.

The illustrations and directions that follow should guide you to the approximate location of each point. From there, it will be simply a matter of probing with your thumbnails until you hit the target.

Chapter 10

46 BODY POINTS: THE KNEE POINTS

POINT KNEE 1

Chinese Name: Liang-Ch'iu
English Translation: Beam Mound
Comments: *Point Knee 1* is among the easiest points to reach, and it often signals its location by being exceptionally tender. Those are two reasons why I have chosen to start with it. Moreover, this point may be the only body point many people will need to stimulate. It is especially effective in relieving backache that travels into the thigh.

Location: The point is exactly two finger widths above the upper, outer border of the kneecap or patella (see Fig. 5). There is a small depression at this spot. Dig your thumbnail into the depression, and you should feel a peculiar sensation travelling up your thigh.

If you have trouble locating it, try the following approach. Sit down, with the left leg straight, and rest your right palm on your left kneecap as shown in Fig. 6. *Point Knee 1* will be approximately where your bent thumbtip rests. To find the matching point above the other knee, of course, you reverse the procedure.

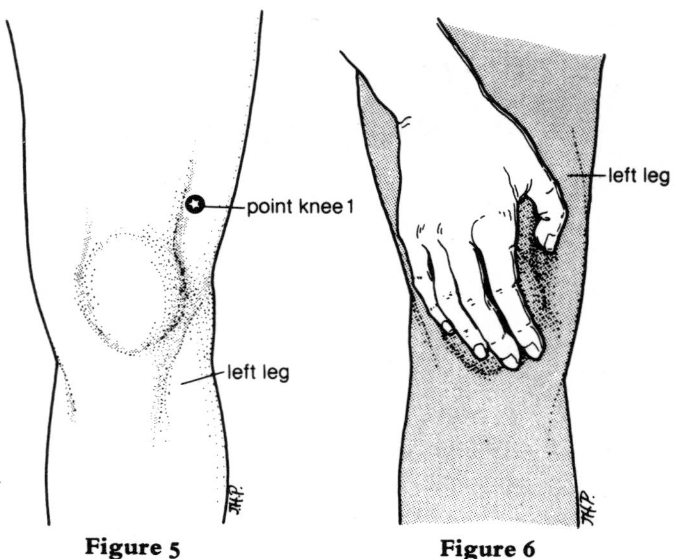

Figure 5 **Figure 6**

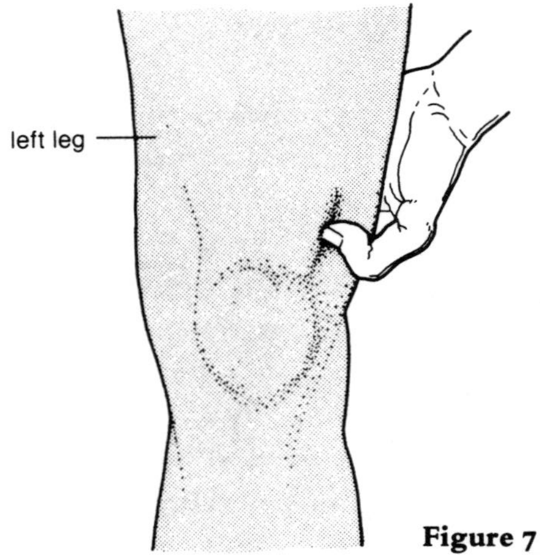

Figure 7

Stimulation: *Point Knee 1* is stimulated by pressing the fingers into the underside of the thigh. Bend your thumb and press the thumbnail into *Point Knee 1*, as is shown in Fig. 7.

POINT KNEE 2

Chinese Name: Hsueh-Hai
English Translation: Sea of Blood
Comments: Simultaneous pressure on *Point Knee 1* and *Point Knee 2* often produces very effective backache relief. In many cases, no other points are needed.

Location: This point is on the other side of the kneecap from *Point Knee 1*, on the medial or inward side of the leg. Exactly two finger widths above the upper, inner border of the kneecap is a depression, and in that depression lies *Point Knee 2* (see Fig. 8).

To guide yourself to the approximate location, sit down as before, but this time put your right palm over your right kneecap, as shown in Fig. 9. *Point Knee 2* is roughly where your bent thumbtip rests.

This point, too, is often exquisitely tender during backache episodes. You may find it highly sensitive at other times as well. Many people are quite ticklish when clutched simultaneously at the *Point Knee 1* and *Point Knee 2* locations.

Stimulation: To stimulate both points simultaneously, use both thumbnails first on one knee, then on the other. Fig. 10 shows how to exert maximum thumbnail pressure on these two points. Wrap your fingers under your thigh and squeeze.

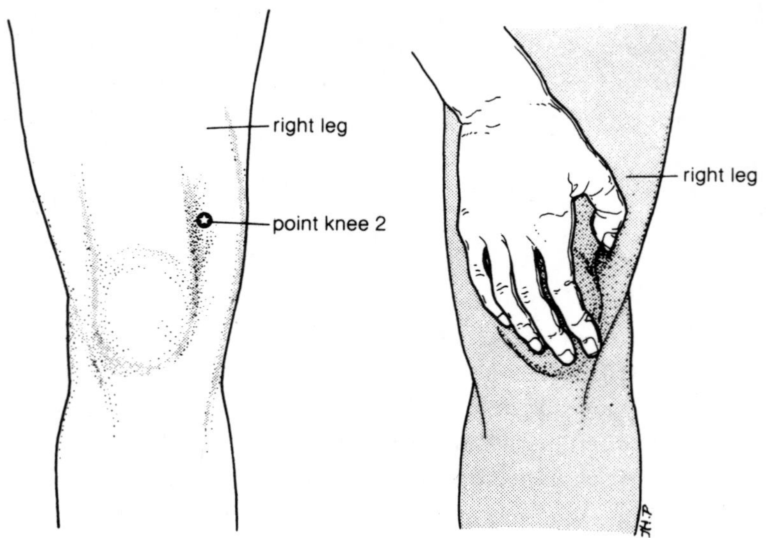

Figure 8

Figure 9

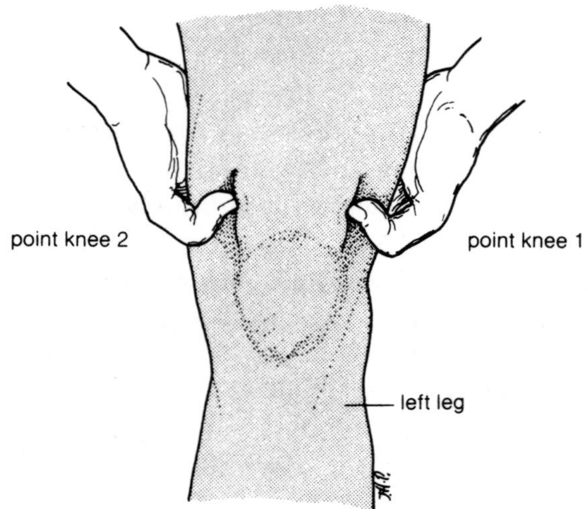

Figure 10

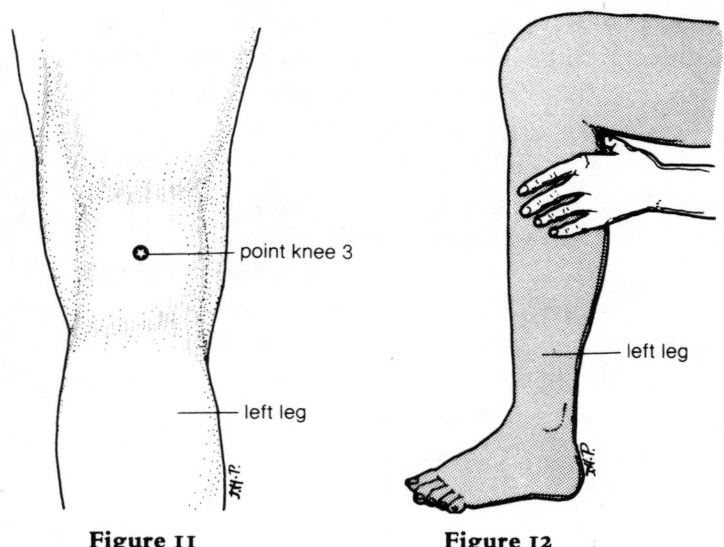

Figure 11 **Figure 12**

POINT KNEE 3

Chinese Name: Wei-Chung

English translation: Commanding Median

Comments: *Point Knee 3* is especially useful for relieving pains in the thigh and calf. As with the other knee points, it may be the only body point that you need to stimulate.

Location: The point is behind the knee. It is exactly in the middle of the popliteal transverse crease, the fold at the back of your knee joint (see Fig. 11). Like the other two knee loci, *Point Knee 3* is often sensitive. You can find it by probing along the popliteal crease with your thumbnail until you hit a spot that sends odd sensations down your leg.

Stimulation: This locus is easy to stimulate. Some

people find it more natural to stimulate the right locus with the right hand, the left with the left. Others find that they feel more comfortable crossing over and stimulating each point with the opposite-sided hand. Either way, your fingers should be on the front of your leg, knee bent, just below the knee (Fig. 12), to help your bent thumb apply the necessary force.

If you wish, you can reinforce one hand with the other. Or, if you find that you can obtain good results with just one-handed pressure, you can stimulate both *Point Knee 3* points simultaneously.

Chapter 11
BODY POINTS: THE ANKLE POINT

THE ANKLE POINT

Chinese Name: K'un-lun

English Translation: K'un Lun Mountains

Comments: *The Ankle Point* is especially effective in relieving back pains that radiate down the leg. In combination with *Point Thigh 1* (or with *Points Thigh 1* and *2*, see Figs. 20–24), it may be the only body point you need to stimulate. Some people will find that just stimulating *The Ankle Point* provides sufficient pain relief for leg and backaches.

Location: This point is on the outer side of your ankle. The large bony protuberance there, the lower end of the fibula or outer leg bone, is called the lateral malleolus. Rearward from the malleolus, between it and the heel cord (the calcaneus or Achilles tendon), is a large, almost bowl-shaped depression. *The Ankle Point* is in that depression, precisely in its centre, at the same level as the tip of the lateral malleolus (see Fig. 13).

Stimulation: There are two ways to stimulate this point. Some people find they can exert effective pressure by putting the fingers under the heel (Fig. 14).

Most, however, seem to get stronger action with the fingers around the back of the heel cord and behind the inner side of the ankle (see Fig. 15).

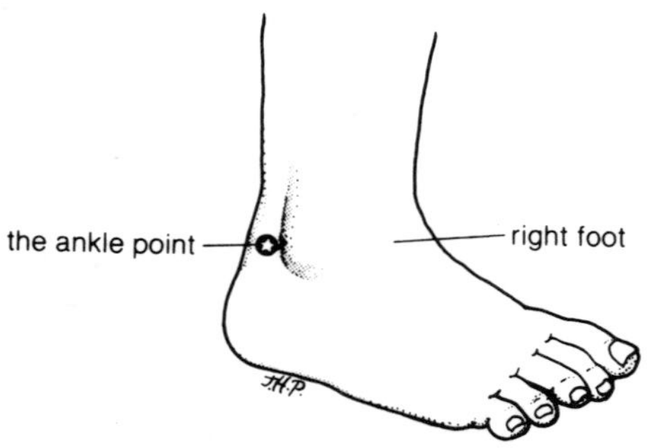

Figure 13

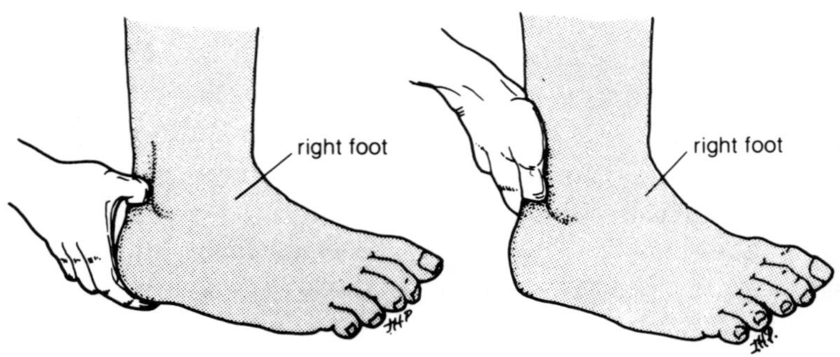

Figure 14 **Figure 15**

Chapter 12
BODY POINTS: THE BACK POINTS

POINT BACK 1

Chinese Name: Ta Ch'ang Shu

English Translation: Large Intestine Locus

Comments: It is possible to use *Point Back 1* in public without drawing attention to yourself. Using the hands-on-hips technique, the points can be stimulated while the person appears quite natural. It is an excellent point to use to alleviate back strain while sitting.

Location: This is among the more difficult points for most people to locate, so you may need to do somewhat more probing than was necessary with the easily found knee and ankle points. Remember to be alert for the phenomenon of 'travelling' sensation that lets you know you are on target. If you have trouble finding the point, it may make its presence known more clearly when you next suffer from backache.

The point (Fig. 16) is in the lumbar region of the back, 1½ finger inches out from the centre of the spine on each side. If you run your fingers up your spine, the bony knobs that you feel are the rearward-projecting spinous processes of the vertebrae. The tips of these

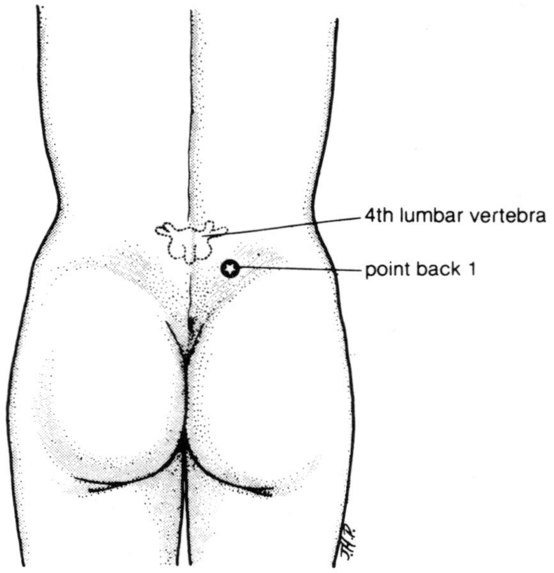

Figure 16

spinous processes mark the exact centre of the back.

Measuring sideways 1½ finger inches from the spinous processes will help you fix the lateral position of *Point Back 1*. Finding the vertical position will be harder.

The point is near the spinous process of the fourth lumbar vertebra. It is slightly lower than the top of the ilium with the thumbs extending horizontally back towards the spine, as shown in Fig. 17. The *Back 1* pair of points should be roughly where your thumbtips rest. Probe the area until you find a small depression, remembering not to go closer to your spine than a finger inch and a half. *Point Back 1* is in the depression.

Stimulation: The *Back 1* points can be stimulated simultaneously on both sides, using the same position

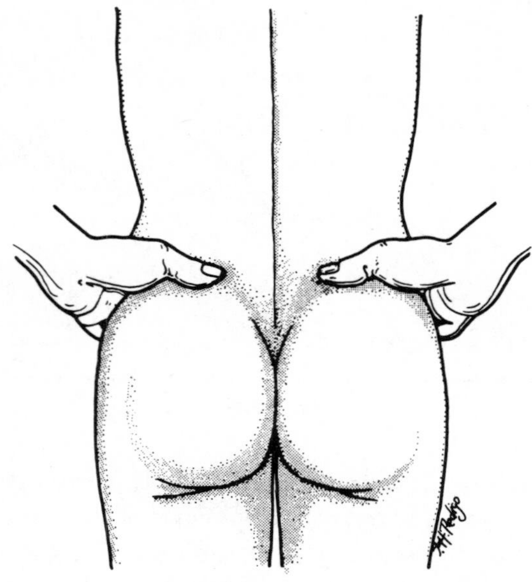

Figure 17

for finding the point. The hands-on-hips position allows for strong, sustained pressure.

POINT BACK 2

Chinese Name: Huan-T'iao

English Translation: Circular Jump

Comments: *Point Back 2* is highly effective for relieving sciatic pain. Some people may find that this point alone is sufficient for relief from sciatica.

Location: This point is lower on the back than *Point Back 1*. It is found at the top of the buttocks. As Fig. 18 shows, it is in between the sacrum (the bone that anchors

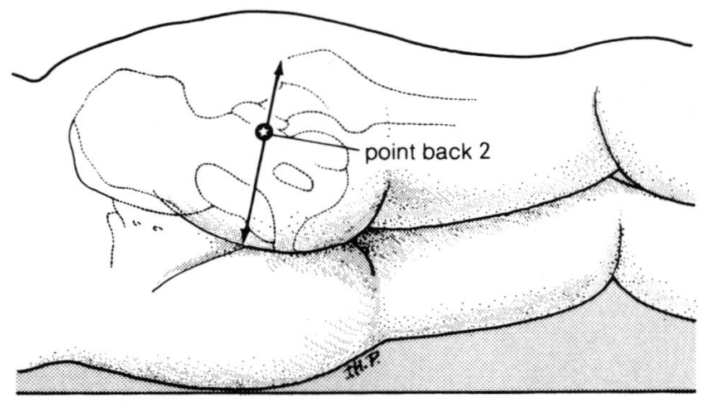

Figure 18

the spine into the pelvic girdle) and the greater trochanter (the large knob near the upper end of the thighbone).

To find this point, you must first find the greater trochanter. The ilium is the hipbone. It is the top and side of the pelvic girdle, the great bone on which your belt rests. The greater trochanter is a good deal lower.

Stand up and put the heel of your hand on your hipbone, with the fingers extending straight down the side of your leg. Move your leg back and forth and from side to side. You should feel a large, round bony knob moving under your fingertips. That is the greater trochanter. This bony protuberance is on the outerside of the thighbone (femur) and slightly below where the rounded end of the femur fits into its hip socket.

To find *Point Back 2*, lie down on your left side with your knees drawn up comfortably. Do not cramp your knees against your chest. Find the greater trochanter with your fingers. Then slide your thumb around your back until you find your sacrum; it is the large, flat prominence between the base of the spine and the tailbone. In most people, the outline of the sacrum is fairly easy to feel. If you have trouble, you may find the sacrum more easily by moving your hips. The sacroiliac joint is not very flexible. However, it is sometimes possible to feel some movement between the sacrum and the pelvic bone on either side.

Now estimate the distance between the trochanter and the nearest edge of the sacrum. *Point Back 2* is closer to the trochanter, about one-third of the distance from that bony knob to the sacrum.

Stimulation: *Point Back 2* is stimulated by wrapping the fingers around the thighbone (femur). The hand is extended and the bent thumb is positioned to apply pressure to *Point Back 2* (Fig. 19).

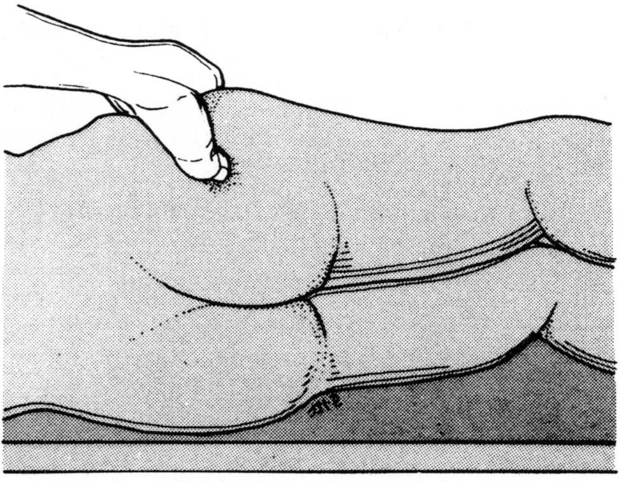

Figure 19

Chapter 13
BODY POINTS: THE THIGH POINTS

POINT THIGH 1

Chinese Name: Fung-Shih
English Translation: Windy Fair
Comments: *Point Thigh 1* can be stimulated without appearing unnatural, if you are seated at a desk or table. It is also a convenient point to stimulate for backache that occurs while seated.

Location: On the outside of your thigh is a long 'valley' between two large muscles, the biceps femoris and the vastus lateralis. *Point Thigh 1* is in that valley on the outside of the thigh. It is 7 finger inches higher than the popliteal crease at the back of the knee (Fig. 20).

An easy way for most people to locate it is to stand at attention with your hands flat against the outsides of your thighs. *Point Thigh 1* will be near the tip of each middle finger (Fig. 21).

Stimulation: Once you find it and are sure of its location, you may find you can stimulate it most easily with your bent thumbs while seated. The point can be pressed bilaterally with the fingers wrapped around the under-surface of the thighs for extra leverage (Fig. 22).

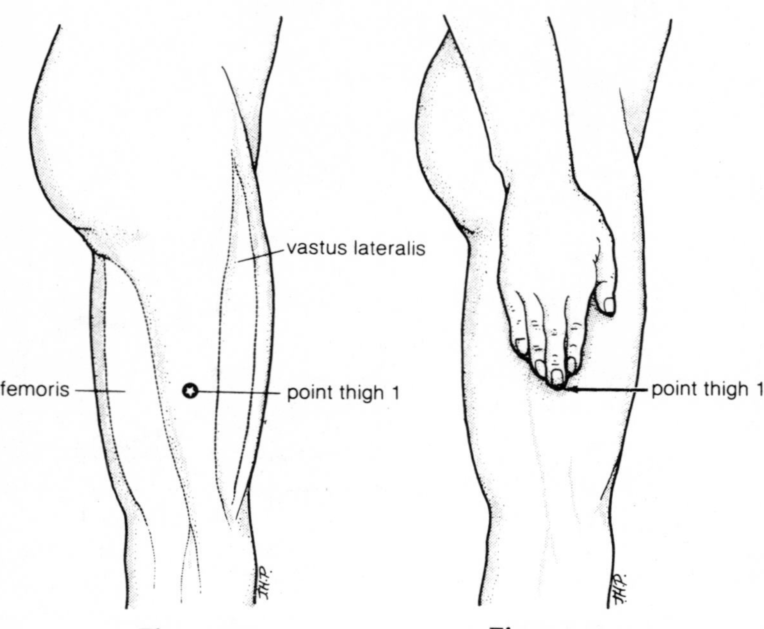

Figure 20

Figure 21

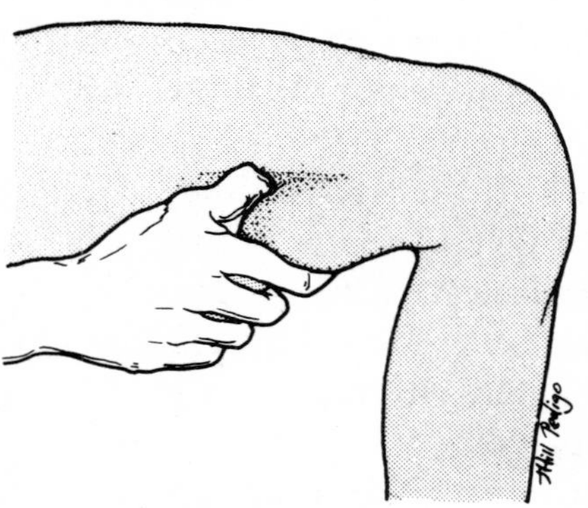

Figure 22

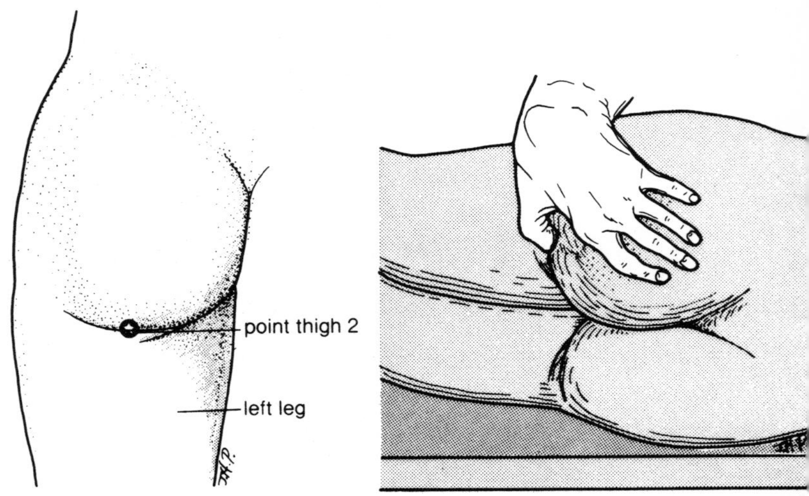

Figure 23

Figure 24

POINT THIGH 2

Chinese Name: Cheng-Fu

English Translation: Support

Comments: *Point Thigh 2* is one of the very easiest to find. It is also one of the most effective for relief of backache that travels into the buttock.

Location: It is exactly in the middle of the gluteal fold, the crease under each buttock (Fig. 23).

Stimulation: Most people find it easiest to stimulate *Point Thigh 2* one side at a time. Lie on your side. Press the upper point with the upper thumbnail (Fig. 24). If you are lying on your right side, press the point under the left buttock with the thumb of your left hand. Your fingers should be on the upper portion of the buttock.

Chapter 14
BODY POINTS: THE LOWER LEG POINT

THE LOWER LEG POINT

Chinese Name: Ch'eng-Shan
English Translation: Supporting Hill
Comments: *The Lower Leg Point* is easy to find and easy to stimulate. It is particularly effective for sciatic pain. This radiates down into the leg from the sciatic nerve in the lower back and sometimes travels as far as the foot.

Location: The back of your lower leg, or calf, is shaped by a long muscle called the gastrocnemius. It is anchored by the Achilles tendon at its lower end, and above that it divides into two bands of 'heads'. You can feel a groove between the two heads, precisely in the middle of your calf at its widest point. If you have trouble locating the groove, a good way to find it is to stand on tiptoe to tense the muscle and make it more prominent. The groove should then be deeper and thus easier to find.

The Lower Leg Point is at the lower end of the muscle groove, 8 finger inches below the popliteal (knee) crease (Fig. 25).

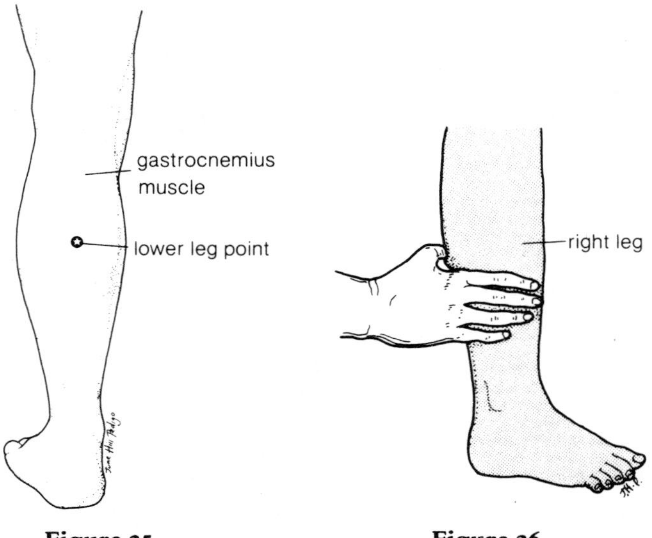

Figure 25

Figure 26

Stimulation: The locus can be stimulated on both sides at one time. Put the nail of your bent thumb in the point, and apply opposing pressure with your fingers on your shinbone (Fig. 26).

Chapter 15
BODY POINTS: A REVIEW

If you have studied the last five chapters, you have learned how to locate and stimulate nine pairs of body points. As we explained in Chapter 8, most people find it necessary to stimulate only one or two body points, or pairs of body points. Many people will now find it helpful to review the basic principles of relieving backaches that we discussed in Chapter 8. Those include the following:

1. Preparation before starting auto-acupressure
   a. Diagnosis of problem
   b. Re-evaluation of drug regimens
2. The thumbnail technique
3. Use of muscle leverage
4. Amount of pressure necessary
5. How long to press
6. Choosing auto-acupressure points
   a. Which are most effective
   b. Which are easiest to stimulate
7. Pairing of points
8. Repeat applications
9. Body position during point stimulation

When you feel that you have a working knowledge of the system of body points, you are ready to learn about the ear point system. Many people find that stimulating a single ear point, or pair of ear points, brings relief from backache. Others may find that stimulating the combination of a single ear point and a single body point produces quick and significant relief from backache.

In the next chapter, we will study the basic principles of relieving back pains with the auto-acupressure system of ear points.

Chapter 16
EAR POINTS: BASIC PRINCIPLES

Western medical researchers and Oriental acupuncturists have observed a highly consistent pattern of connections between various points in the ears and corresponding body parts. Every part of the body is represented: the head, the trunk, the limbs and extremities. It is possible to draw a schematic map of the entire body in the two pinnae; it would show that certain parts of the ears contain neural connections with the hands, certain parts with the hips, and so on. This tracery of nerves in the ears is a miniaturized reflection of certain nerve pathways in the body as a whole.

The existence of such a convenient ear point system is one good reason for attacking a backache through the ears. Another reason is that the nerves of the ear point system are peculiarly accessible to thumbnail pressure. The external ears are built mainly of thin cartilage covered with skin. They ordinarily contain no bone, and most parts of the ear contain no muscle. In many other parts of the body, nerves are often hidden behind bone or buried in deep masses of muscle and other tissue. There is no convenient way to stimulate them. However, in the pinnae, the nerves are easily accessible and so can be stimulated without difficulty.

The ear point system can be used before, after, or in conjunction with the body point system, or the ear point system can be used alone. Many people find that the ear point system gives them excellent relief most of the time. They use the body point system less often; sometimes, only when their pain is more than usually severe. Others find that certain combinations of the two systems work best for them.

I suggest that you experiment in the following way when you are next troubled by a backache. Try the ear point system first. If it gives you only partial relief, try those body points that you have found to be the most effective for you.

That combination may give you effective, long-lasting relief. However, some people find that reversing the combination works better for them. They use the body point system for *initial* relief, as at the beginning of an arduous day. Then use the ear point system for *maintenance* of the effects throughout the day.

An advantage of the ear point system is that you can use it at any time of day. You can use it in any situation, in public or in private. Some of the body point system points require that you partially undress, lie down, or adopt somewhat awkward positions. Consequently, it is not always possible to stimulate some of the body points in the middle of a busy day. Some of those points can be pressed unobtrusively while sitting in a chair, but others cannot. Thus you may find the ear point system highly useful. If a backache is troubling you while you are at work, at a social gathering, or riding in a car, you can stimulate the ear points unobtrusively. To other people, you will look as though you are only toying with your ears, a perfectly natural human gesture. (Your thumbnail may leave a red mark. However, it should not be very noticeable and should vanish in minutes.)

STIMULATION

In stimulating the ear points, be guided in general by the directions I gave in Chapter 8, dealing with the body point system. The stimulation techniques for both systems are substantially the same.

Use your thumbnail, with the thumb bent as shown in Fig. 1. With most points, to give the thumbnail something to press against, you can put your forefinger on the other side of the ear for a pincerlike squeezing action. Press hard enough to make the point under your thumbnail hurt mildly. As with the body point system, you can use either steady pressure or rhythmic off-on pressure. Maintain it for 30 seconds.

As I warned before, it is dangerous to apply auto-acupressure with long or pointed thumbnails. The nails should be short and rounded. It is never necessary in auto-acupressure to pierce the skin or to leave any injury beyond a temporary red mark.

WHICH EAR?

If your back pain is centred or diffuse, not clearly one-sided, then you will generally find it most effective to press paired points on both ears.

If the pain is one-sided, one ear may well be sufficient. Often, in the case of one-sided pain, you will find that certain points on one ear are markedly more tender than the corresponding points on the other ear. Do not assume, however, that the tender ear will always be on the same side of the body as the back, buttock, or leg pain. Under some circumstances, you will find that the opposite-sided ear is the more tender.

Thus, when your back aches, you will need to explore your ears for tenderness. As with the body point system, the greatest pain-relieving effect always comes from stimulating the most tender points.

Chapter 17
EAR POINTS: STRUCTURE OF THE EAR

In medical terminology, the external ear is called the auricula or pinna. It is richly endowed with a highly complex network of fine but amazingly sensitive nerves. They interconnect through many neural pathways with nerves in distant parts of the body. When they are stimulated properly with either a needle or a thumbnail, they can produce astonishingly powerful effects in those distant parts. You are soon to discover the effects on pain in the back, buttocks, and legs.

In the next chapter, with words and drawings, I will guide you through the ear point system. You will learn points that are relevant to back pains and to the sciatic pains and leg pains that are often their unwelcome companion. But first, as we did with the body point system, I will need to give you some instruction on basic anatomy.

EXPLORING YOUR EARS

If you look closely at your ears in a mirror, you will probably see that they are not shaped precisely alike. In some people, the difference is immediately apparent, while in others, it is subtle: a more pronounced curve here, a longer groove there. Ears are remarkably variable, even on the same head.

They are still more variable from one person to another. The size, the degree of protrusion, the colour, the shapes of various parts of the structure vary wildly. This is even true in members of the same family.

The ear changes shape and texture continually through life. A child's ear cartilage is soft and very pliable. As he ages, it will grow harder and less elastic. Some parts may wrinkle; the lobe may grow longer; hair may appear on the top and elsewhere. If the ear has been subjected to a lot of trauma in its lifetime, there may be some fairly gross changes and distortions. The 'cauliflower ear' of a boxer is an exaggerated example. Ears that have been frequently exposed to severe cold or to sunburn may also become more than normally thickened.

But despite all these variations, the basic design of the human pinna remains constant from one head to another. If you look at Fig. 27, you will see a drawing of an ear with the prominent parts named. You will need to know the names of these parts to follow the directions in the next chapter. Study the drawing and identify the parts on your own ears by exploring them with thumb and forefinger. There are not many of them. Some of the names are appealingly imaginative. To help you in your exploration, I will supplement the drawing by describing the parts in words:

The large central cavity is called the *concha*, from a Greek word meaning seashell.

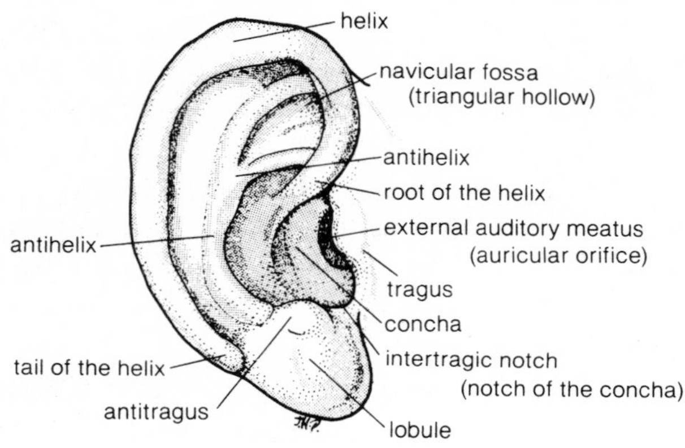

Figure 27

The ear-canal hole in the concha is called the *auricular orifice* or the *external auditory meatus*.

Directly in front of the meatus and partly covering it is a prominent little knob of cartilage called the *tragus*. In some people the tragus has, on its underside, a tuft of hair something like a goat's beard. The name literally means he-goat.

Across the concha from the tragus, and separated from it by a small notch, is another outcropping of cartilage called the *antitragus*. The notch is called the *intertragic notch* or simply the *notch of the concha*.

Below the antitragus is the lobe; in medical terminology it is called the *lobule*. It contains no cartilage. From ancient times, it has been used by both men and women as a place from which to hang rings and other decorations. In some people, the lobe is securely attached to the neighbouring facial skin near the angle of the jaw. In others it is clearly separate. This is an oddity of heredity and is linked to certain other inherited traits.

The prominent outer rim of the ear is called the *helix*. Follow it on your own ear with thumb and finger and you will notice that it starts just above the lobe. This is the so-called *tail* of the helix. The helix then runs up the side of the ear, over the top, and down into the concha. This part of the helix, where it runs backwards across the bowl of the concha, is called the *root* or *crus* (rhymes with 'loose'). The crus of the helix divides the concha into two unequal parts.

Inside the helix, running parallel with it for a short distance, is another ridge called the *antihelix*. Towards the top of the ear the antihelix divides into two ridges or *crura*. Both ridges then disappear under the helix. Between these two crura is a shallow triangular depression which is named the *navicular fossa*. *Navicular* means boat-shaped, and *fossa* comes from a word meaning ditch. For simplicity, I will refer to this area from now on as the *triangular hollow*.

Now, while you remember the basic structure of the external ear, it is the time to learn how to relieve back pains with the ear point system.

Chapter 18
EAR POINTS: METHODS OF LOCATION AND STIMULATION

To find these points, you will have to use, in miniature, a technique you learned in Chapter 9. Each point has a peculiarly tender feeling, and when you feel it, that is the signal that you are on target. As we go through the points, I will describe each as closely as I can. You should also refer to Fig. 26 for further guidance. But the final targeting will be up to you. Put your thumbnail in the approximate location of each point; then move it back and forth, by the smallest possible increments, until you touch the tender spot for which you are looking.

If you have trouble finding the points under ordinary conditions, wait until your next attack of backache. It is likely that some, or all, of the points will then become considerably more tender.

THE STARTING POINT

As Fig. 28 shows, this is on the root or crus of the helix as it exits from the concha. In many people, there is a fairly deep crosswise notch in the crus at this point,

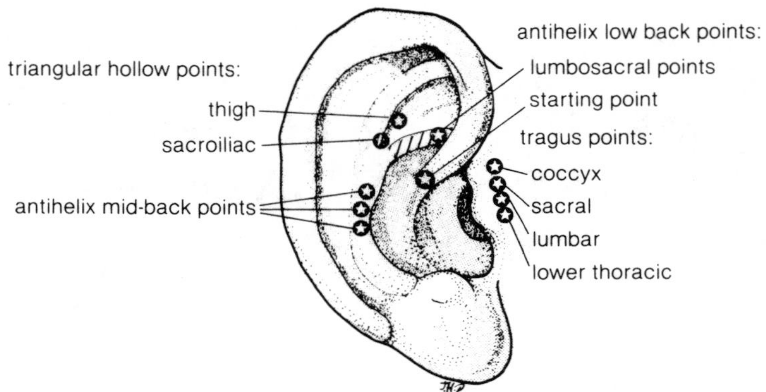

Figure 28

much like a notch in a long mountain ridge. Other people will find a tiny knob of cartilage just behind the point. Probe with your thumbnail until you feel this often tender spot. During episodes of backache, it may become exquisitely tender.

It is called the *Starting Point* because it is probably the easiest of all microsystem points to find. You may want to experiment with it before going on to the other points. Stimulating this point may produce excellent relief of lumbar and sciatic pain. Some people find that it is usually the only microsystem point they need.

Some find that they can stimulate this point well by putting the forefinger behind the ear and squeezing against the thumbnail. In most people, however, the ear is attached to the head in such a way that it is hard to get the forefinger into the right position. If you find that this is the case with you, stimulate the point by pressing directly inwards against your head (Fig. 29).

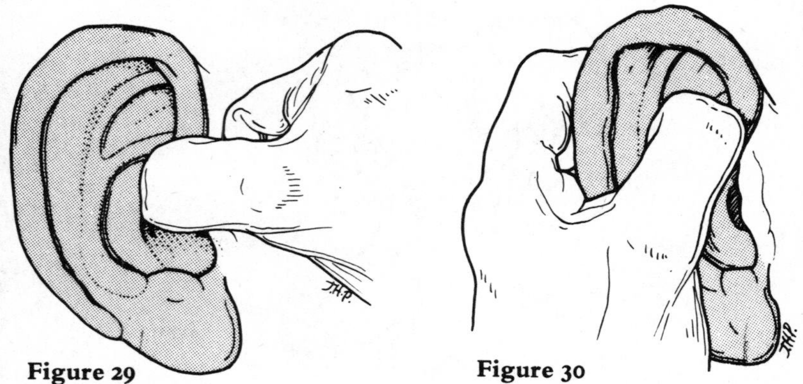

Figure 29 **Figure 30**

THE ANTIHELIX LOW BACK POINTS

The positions of these points vary from person to person and from time to time in the same person, depending on the exact nature and location of the back disorder. As Fig. 28 shows, the *Antihelix Low Back Points* lie along the lower ridge of the antihelix, starting at the place where the two ridges form a fork (the apex of the triangular hollow) and ending where the lower ridge disappears under the overlying helix.

When you have pain in the lower back or sacroiliac area, probe along that antihelix ridge with your thumbnail until you find the most tender point. Start by lifting the overlying helix and probing under it. Then very slowly work your way back to the fork of the antihelix.

To stimulate this point effectively, form pincers with your thumb and forefinger. The thumbnail should press directly into the point on the outer surface of your ear, while the fingernail presses the same point from behind (Fig. 30).

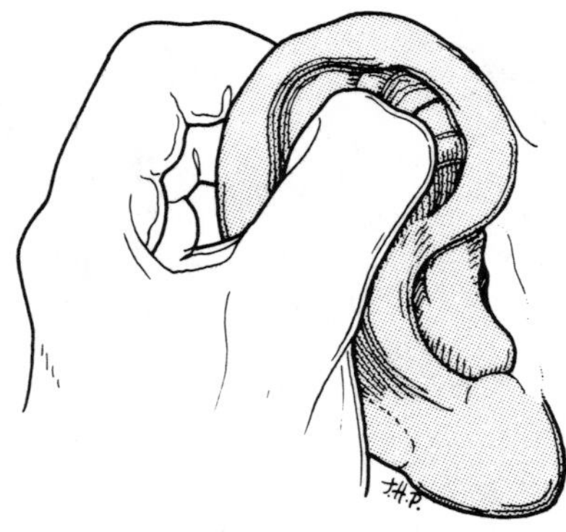

Figure 31

THE TRIANGULAR HOLLOW POINTS

Points relating to the lower back are in the lower, rearward part of the triangular hollow. They are near the fork of the two antihelix ridges (see Fig. 28). As before, you should probe with your thumbnail in very small increments until you find unusual tenderness.

These points, when well stimulated, relieve pain and spasm in the region of the sacroiliac, the buttocks, and the thighs. They can be stimulated effectively with the thumb-and-forefinger pincers (Fig. 31).

THE ANTIHELIX MID-BACK POINTS

These points are on the antihelix, at or above the place where the crus of the helix abuts against it (Fig. 28). When stimulated correctly, a tender point in this area relieves pain and spasm in the thoracic or mid-back region.

The point can be stimulated, like the others, with the thumbnail on the outer ear surface and the nail of the forefinger behind it.

THE TRAGUS POINT

Use this point for chronic backache if you fail to get adequate relief from the points we have already studied. As Fig. 28 shows, the point is near the top and towards the front of the tragus. It is just behind the place (marked on some people by a faint groove) where the tragus joins the side of the face. In most people, the point is directly in front of the meatus (the opening of the ear canal).

This point is unlike all the others in one very important respect. It is never necessary to stimulate the point

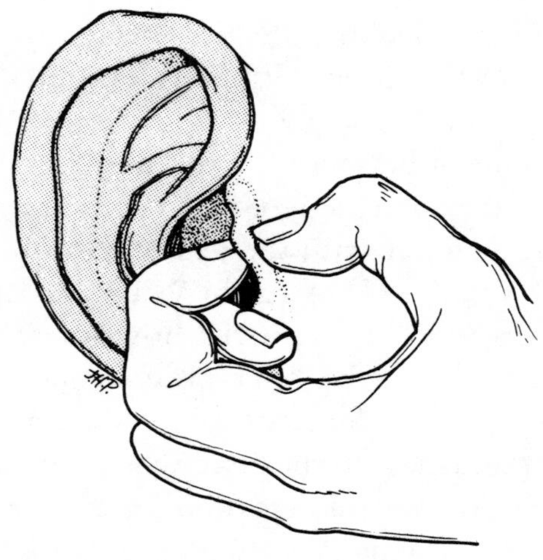

Figure 32

on both ears. Instead, utilize the following procedure:

If you are right-handed, stimulate the left tragus. If you are left-handed, stimulate the right. This somewhat mysterious-sounding rule is dictated by a peculiarity of the nervous system. The tragus opposite the hand-favoured side is always the one with the clearest neural connections with the spine.

Most people find it comfortable to stimulate the *Tragus Point* with the favoured hand. That is, if you are right-handed, stimulate the left point with your right hand. Hold the tragus between thumbnail and fore-finger so that the thumbnail is vertical. Be careful not to let your forefingernail slip into the ear-canal opening (Fig. 32).

THE CONCHA POINT

This point, unlike the others, is behind the ear rather than on its outer surface. Study its location carefully in Fig. 33.

To find the point, put your forefinger in the concha, just above the intertragic notch. Your thumb should be behind your ear with the pad of the thumb resting against the back of the lobe. With the tip of your thumb, you will feel a convex bowl of cartilage, the underside of the concha. Now probe with your thumb-nail near the lower, inner corner of the cartilage, close to the lobe and close to the place where the ear joins the neck (Fig. 34). You should find an extremely tender point there, particularly during episodes of pain in the lower back.

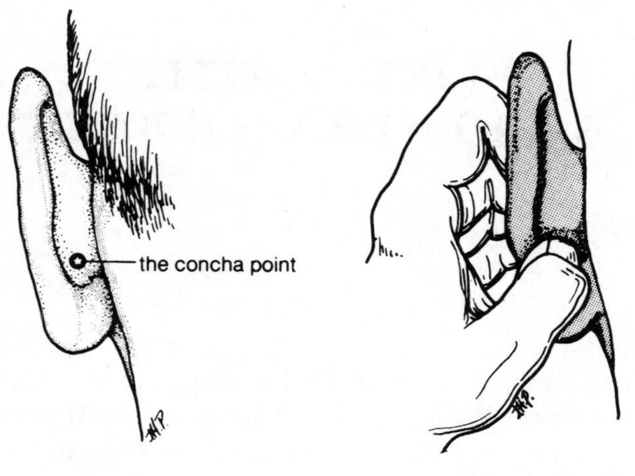

Figure 33 **Figure 34**

The point corresponds to the lower part of the spine. Many people find it highly effective when used after one of the *Antihelix Low Back Points.*

Once you have learned to locate and stimulate the ear points, you should select your favourite point or two. During your next episode of backache, try the ear point system first. Then try it in combination with your favourite body point.

Now that you know how to relieve your backaches, it is wise to learn how to prevent them. The next chapter will advise you on how to live with a back that is vulnerable to pain.

Chapter 19
LIVING WITH A VULNERABLE BACK

A vulnerable back is one that is subject to frequent or chronic pain. As we saw in Chapters 5, 6, and 7, there are a variety of possible reasons for such pain. In Chapters 8–18, we learned how to relieve backache with the Auto-Acupressure Systems of Body Points and Ear Points. This chapter will advise you on other precautionary measures to reduce the frequency and severity of painful episodes.

EXERCISE

This is one topic on which you should most certainly consult your doctor. Certain exercises can aggravate a back problem instead of alleviating it. That is why I do not intend to prescribe exercises in this book. Only a doctor who is familiar with your entire health status will know whether a given exercise would be beneficial, dangerous, or useless to you.

In most cases, people with vulnerable backs are encouraged to exercise daily so as to strengthen muscles of the abdomen, the back, and the buttocks. These are the muscle areas that do the major work of holding the spine erect and maintaining the proper curvatures. If you allow your abdominal muscles to become weak, the ultimate result could be a protruding abdomen that might produce a sway-backed posture (lordosis) which will put damaging stress on the lumbar area of your spine. The muscles of the back itself do the main work of supporting the upper part of the spine. The large buttock muscles help hold the upper body in proper alignment with hips and legs.

In many cases, a doctor will suggest calisthenics such as bent-knee and pelvic-tilt sit-ups, designed to demand strenuous exertion of certain specific muscle groups. However, such exercises are hard work and are boring. The unfortunate truth is that only a minority of people actually perform them religiously over a span of years. Thus, many doctors simply counsel back patients to get plenty of general exercise in some activity they enjoy, such as swimming, walking, bicycling, etc. It can certainly be stated as a general truth that your chances of avoiding back problems grow very much better as you improve your muscle tone and strength, your posture, and other aspects of your general health.

BODY WEIGHT

Try to keep your weight within the normal tolerances for a man or woman of your height. It is obvious that a heavy upper body will put more than normal stress on the spine as it tries to hold up all that weight.

But if you are now overweight, beware of fad dieting

or any attempt to shed pounds in too great a hurry. As we saw in an earlier chapter, poor nutrition can aggravate certain back disorders. It can even become one of their basic causes. There are safe and unsafe ways to lose weight. In your local library, you will find books devoted to both ways. Ask your doctor to recommend one of the safe ones.

SITTING

Favour straight-backed, firm chairs, not heavily padded ones. The body sinks too deeply into thick padding, causing excessive flexure of the spine.

When you sit, try to have one or both knees higher than your hips. This is the sitting position that puts the least strain on the spine. Crossing your legs will lift one knee high. Or you can lift both knees by putting your feet on a low stool. However, be sure your knees are bent, so that your feet rest on their soles. Do not extend your legs straight out so that your feet rest on the backs of the heels. That position increases strain on the back.

To improve your sitting posture when driving a car, pull the seat forward enough to lift your knees high. When riding as a passenger, cross your legs or put one foot on the transmission hump. You may find that car seats are too deeply padded for you, and that you develop pain and stiffness on trips that are not especially long. If so, you may get relief from a special straight-backed car seat. Such seats are made to fit over the standard padded seats. They can be bought at medical supply houses and some department stores.

UNUSUALLY HEAVY STRESS

You may know in advance that you must endure a particularly stressful day. For example, you must take a long automobile trip and then unload heavy suitcases from the car. You know from past experience that this will produce backache. In a case such as this, ask your doctor beforehand if he can recommend temporary help. He may prescribe a back brace or orthopaedic corset. Such a device can help you through a period of unusually heavy back stress. In these special situations, it may help you avoid new back damage.

An orthopaedic appliance such as a back brace should be looked upon only as a temporary aid. Remove it as soon as you and your doctor feel it is safe to do so. You should beware of becoming dependent on it. If you lapse into the habit of wearing it every day, you could dangerously weaken your back and the muscles that support it.

CAR DOORS

One very common body movement that can cause pain, and even acute trauma when awkwardly done, is that of climbing in and out of a car. The action of ducking the head while twisting the body is hard to carry out gracefully.

A good procedure is to get in and out of the car much as you would get in and out of bed. When entering the car, first sit sideways on the edge of the seat, with your feet outside on the ground. Then lean back so that your head clears the doorway and enters the car. Finally, swing your legs inside. To climb out, reverse the process: first swing your feet sideways and out onto the ground, and then lean forward enough to stand.

STANDING

If you must stand still for a long time, try to rest one foot higher than the other. If you are working on a ladder, put one foot on a rung higher than the other. If you are waiting at an airport or railway station, rest one foot on your suitcase.

This standing position puts the least possible strain on the back. Tavernkeepers all over the world are aware of this. At almost any bar where the patrons stand, there is a rail on which they can rest one foot. Utilizing the bar rail with occasional changes in position, many people find it is possible to stand for several hours without discomfort. By contrast, an uncomfortable experience for most backache sufferers is a cocktail party where one must spend a long time standing with both feet flat on the floor. In such situations, you will probably find it helpful to straighten the back while standing. You can do so by tilting the pelvis. To further reduce strain, bend one knee, and keep the other knee straight.

BENDING AND LIFTING

When you bend to pick something up, you should bend your knees as well as your back. It is easier on your back either to crouch down on both legs or rest on one knee only. When working with something on the ground, it is better to bend down on one knee rather than on both.

If you carry a heavy weight for any distance, carry it close to your body with your elbows bent, not straight. Even with bent elbows, it is hazardous to lift a heavy weight higher than shoulder level. If you are carrying some heavy or awkward object with another person, be sure that both of you lift it and put it down together, as a team. If the other person drops his or her end, drop yours too. Trying to catch a heavy weight in that manner can do serious damage to your back. It is better to break a piece of furniture than a vertebra.

When carrying anything heavy, do not twist your body. If you must turn while heavily burdened, turn with your feet.

Avoid lifting heavy objects that are in tight, awkward places. Be especially careful with objects so situated that you cannot get your feet under the weight. You will recall that I injured my own back once when trying to lift a sack of lawn fertilizer from a car boot. The standard boot could hardly have been more ineptly designed; it is hard to think of anything harder on the spine. If you must remove anything heavy from a car boot or any similarly awkward space, either get help or roll the object out. If at all possible, avoid lifting it out.

SLEEPING

People with low backache generally should not lie on their stomachs. For the sake of your back, lie on your side with knees and hips bent. Or lie on your back with a pillow (or rolled blanket or other object) under your knees to bend the knees and hips.

It is best to use a firm, flat mattress. Try to avoid a soft, deep mattress, or an old one with a depression in the middle. Your bed should not allow the middle of your body to sag as in a hammock; it should support your hips firmly, with just enough softness for comfort. If your bed is too soft, you can get relief by putting a bedboard under the mattress.

When travelling, you can get a bedboard on request at many hotels and motels. If that is not possible and if a hotel bed is too soft, make arrangements for someone else to take the mattress off the box spring and put it on the floor. Or you can simply spread blankets on the floor and sleep on them.

FATIGUE

It is best to avoid getting excessively tired during the day. Fatigue can exacerbate many low back problems.

When I was a medical student, I was puzzled one day to see an obstetrician squatting in a crouched position in a hospital corridor. He saw my perplexed look, smiled, and explained that he did this periodically to ease the strain on his back. His work often required him to stand for long periods, bending over an operating table. The squatting position made him feel better in a few minutes.

Anybody with a vulnerable back would do well to emulate that man. Try to find a way of relaxing your back for 5 or 10 minutes, once or twice a day. If possible lie flat on your back on a bed or floor. Elevate your legs on a pillow or cushion so as to exert a mild upward pull on the hips. If you feel pain, you can relieve it with auto-acupressure.

Chapter 20
RELAXATION TECHNIQUES: REST WITHOUT PILLS

Most chronic backache patients rely on some sort of drug to assist sleep. In a recent study at the Mayo Clinic, 65 per cent of patients with chronic pain, not related to malignant tumours, were found to be either drug dependent or drug abusers. In addition to analgesics, tranquillizers, and muscle relaxants, many of my patients have described their prior abuse of sleeping pills and alcoholic beverages to induce sleep. Furthermore, many patients have related to me that they had persistent difficulties with insomnia even after they had learned to relieve their backaches with auto-acupressure. They expressed dissatisfaction with their dependence on pills for sleep, and wanted to 'kick the habit' of drugs for sleep.

The solution I ordinarily offer for such problems involves tapering off unnecessary drugs and substituting a relaxation technique. The brain must sleep. Once pain problems are brought under control, it is ordinarily the inability to relax that delays the onset of sleep.

Because of their sedative effects, relaxation techniques are excellent methods to augment pain relief systems. Being over-anxious, being uptight often causes intensification of both muscle spasm and the subjective discomfort of pain. The more a person's focus turns to the inner awareness of pain, the greater may be the dread of possible destructive effects of pain upon the ability to enjoy and participate in life. Ordinarily, the awareness of pain increases suffering. But there are exceptions. The often quoted observation of wounded soldiers in the battlefield relates the fact that what might otherwise be excruciating pain can be perceived in a positive way. Soldiers with severe wounds have been seen to exhibit euphoria at having earned 'their ticket back home'. In these days of relatively 'cold' rather than 'hot' wars, there are many ferocious 'battles' conducted on athletic fields. It is certainly well known and well documented that sometimes professional and non-professional athletes have played with serious injuries. They were able to overcome pain in the desire for victory.

My acquaintance with relaxation techniques dates back more than three decades ago when I learned techniques of hypnosis. I had the good fortune to witness the use of hypnosis in the treatment of various habit disorders. I was instructed by an excellent hypnotist, who had the ability to induce hypnotic trances in a variety of people. Over two-and-a-half decades ago, I wrote my first monograph on the induction of hypnosis and self-hypnosis. I mention these points to emphasize that I have been able to observe the long-term effectiveness of these techniques over a considerable period of time.

Hypnosis is a state of altered consciousness. It is a condition of heightened awareness of certain stimuli and decreased awareness of others. Hypnosis is better suited for relief of acute pain situations than of chronic pain situations. The use of hypnosis as both an analgesic and an anaesthetic agent has been well documented. Surgical operations have been conducted using hypnosis as the primary anaesthetic.

Currently, I utilize hypnosis in my private office practice for the following particular effects: (1) overcoming memory blocks and resistances in the course of psychotherapy, (2) weight reduction, (3) smoking reduction, and (4) insomnia problems.

Post-hypnotic suggestions may alter a person's behaviour after the cessation of the formal hypnotic state. Post-hypnotic suggestions are utilized in the hypnotic treatment techniques for weight reduction and smoking control. In those cases, the post-hypnotic suggestions given are ordinarily positive ones which encourage the development of aversions to the specific appetites. The treatment of chronic pain may be attempted with a negative post-hypnotic suggestion, such as the absence of awareness. Since denying the awareness of pain is unrealistic, it is not usually a successful method. Positive post-hypnotic suggestions are sometimes beneficial for pain relief. Some patients do respond to associating the perception of pain with pleasant memories and sensations. Again, however, these effects tend to be transient. Ordinarily, they do not produce substantial long-term benefit in most chronic pain patients.

The use of self-hypnosis in insomnia problems is quite helpful for some patients. Nevertheless, it is not a technique which I feel is appropriate for everyone. It requires consultation from a psychiatrist to determine whether self-hypnosis is a desirable procedure. However, a closely related relaxation technique to assist in producing sleep will be offered to you—in detail—at the end of this chapter. Many patients have fallen asleep in my office just in the process of learning it.

Biofeedback is a relaxation technique whereby a person learns to relax muscles which he ordinarily would not have under voluntary control. Biofeedback is a meritorious technique for patients who can learn to use it. Generally, it provides assistance to chronic pain patients and is one of those techniques which can be used to modify pain. Biofeedback is generally able to decrease the perception of some pains by decreasing painful muscle spasm. There are biofeedback instruments available in professional laboratories and available for home use. Your doctor may be able to direct you to someone who can train you in the biofeedback method. Or he may recommend that you buy a biofeedback device to use at home. In brief essence, the biofeedback method would involve the electronic monitoring of a bodily function, such as pulse rate, hand warmth, or muscle movement. If, for example, your low backache caused spasm in the lumbar muscles, electrodes might be attached to those muscles. You could work with the machine until you had developed a state of relaxation in the muscles. Ideally then, you might be able to learn to sit or stand with the same degree of relaxation of your low back muscles as you might obtain at other times when you are lying flat on your back with a pillow under your knees.

Although it was felt that biofeedback might be an answer to many pain problems, long-term follow-up studies simply have not shown that to be the case. Even though one's expectations should be limited, it is again emphasized that this may be a helpful supplementary technique and its use should be considered on advice of your doctor.

Much wisdom about relaxation may be found in the study of yoga. However, the advice of your doctor should be obtained to determine what hatha yoga exercises are prudent for your general state of health and particular back problems. For more than half a century, the pioneer American physician in the field of relaxation techniques has been Dr Edmund Jacobson. His numerous publications include several entire books on progressive relaxation exercises.

As I have already promised, here is the simple relaxation technique which can facilitate the onset of sleep by diminishing anxieties and muscle spasm. This relaxation technique involves the alternate contraction and relaxation of major groups of muscles related to body parts. One starts at the toes and progresses to the head. An example of this effective muscle relaxation technique would be to contract (bend) each set of muscles for 10 to 15 seconds, and then to feel those muscles relax for an equal period of time. To be specific, the relaxation technique would be: bend your toe muscles for 10 seconds. Feel them relax for 10 seconds. Bend the ankle up for 10 seconds. Relax the ankle for 10 seconds. Contract the calf muscles for 10 seconds. Relax the calf muscles for 10 seconds. Contract the thigh muscles for 10 seconds. Relax the thigh muscles for 10 seconds. Contract the abdominal muscles for 10 seconds. Relax the abdominal muscles for 10 seconds. Make a fist for 10 seconds. Relax the fist for 10 seconds. Bend the wrist up for 10 seconds. Relax the wrist for 10 seconds.

Contract the upper arm muscles for 10 seconds. Relax the upper arm muscles for 10 seconds. Shrug the shoulder muscles for 10 seconds. Relax the shoulder muscles for 10 seconds. Tense the neck muscles for 10 seconds. Relax the neck muscles for 10 seconds. Contract the forehead muscles for 10 seconds. Relax the forehead muscles for 10 seconds. Contract the eyelids tightly for 10 seconds. Relax the eyelids for 10 seconds, keeping the eyelids lightly closed. Now feel the state of relaxation that has gone from your toes to your head. Feel the relaxation all the way down the body—from the head to the neck to the shoulder to the arm to the hand to the abdomen to the thigh to the calf to the ankle to the toes.

If performing this relaxation technique has not relaxed you suitably the first time, then repeat it. An alternative technique is to use a longer period of time for each muscle group, such as 15 to 30 seconds. Such relaxation techniques should be encouraged. They are a much healthier, more natural and nontoxic substitute for analgesics, sedative tranquillizers, and sleeping pills.

Our consultation on your backache problems is now almost complete. We have discussed the major aspects of learning to live more comfortably with your illness. We have consulted on diagnoses and treatment methods. We have learned new methods of pain relief. We have discussed how to adapt to the demands of daily living. We have briefly reviewed methods of overcoming anxiety and sleeping problems without drugs. In the next chapter, you may learn how to make your sexual life more fulfilling.

Chapter 21
SEX AND THE BACKACHE PATIENT

One of the most critical problems for backache patients is the loss, or the fear of loss, of sexual function. This problem was typified[7] in a recent study of married patients referred to the pain management centre of the Mayo Clinic. Almost two-thirds of those patients reported impairment in their sexual satisfaction. They stated that sexual intercourse had decreased both in frequency and in quality. Sexual changes, such as these, are very critical life problems. They frequently contribute to deterioration of the overall marital relationship, often resulting in divorce.

A significant percentage of men and women, who did not have sexual difficulties prior to their pain disorders, developed them consequent to their painful state. Frequently occurring sexual problems are difficulties in becoming sexually aroused and in reaching orgasm. Some chronic pain patients lose all interest in sex.

Medication used for pain relief may decrease libido. Tranquillizers, sedatives, and narcotic analgesics all may reduce sexual drive. Corticosteroids may decrease the responses to genital stimulation in both males and females, and in males may induce impotence.

Until very recently, expressions of sexuality or sexual need in physically handicapped people were seen as unusual, if not perverse. Overcoming a person's handicap by obtaining a job or functioning independently are commonly considered praiseworthy achievements. Such praiseworthiness had rarely extended to socially appropriate sexual activity. To most people, the sexual needs of the handicapped individual are considered to vary from humorous to repulsive.

The sexual needs of the physically disabled and chronic pain patients are not identical to those of people in the able-bodied population. People with physical handicaps and chronic pain problems commonly have sexual needs that are accentuated. Their sexual desires are increased by the constant need to be reassured that their disabilities do not repulse their loved ones. Chronic pain patients and physically disabled people usually have an even greater need than other people to prove that their sexual performance can be pleasurable and satisfying.

Medical studies of arthritis patients typify those of all patients with chronic pain problems. Many who have suffered from the severe pain, disfigurement, depression, and prolonged hospitalization associated with arthritis have observed that their sexual relationships became a focus of failure and frustration. As chronic arthritis conditions progressed, close marital relationships often deteriorated. They became guilt laden, overburdened with great emotional strain. Many became devoid of sexual intimacy. Frequently, the results were emotional instability, marital separation, and ultimately divorce.

In the early stages of arthritic disease, women patients with back and hip problems may find that limitation in movement of the hips and other joints makes intercourse painful and therefore unsatisfying. In later stages of arthritic hip disease, traditional positions of intercourse may become impossible. Awareness of the destruction of the body, related to the chronic pain and its resultant depression, may also contribute to the person's loss of sexual function. The loss of sexual pleasure is often the arthritic patient's first significant life loss. It often occurs long before the loss of the ability to walk or the loss of the ability to work.

Low backache and arthritic involvement of the hips are the disabilities most likely to interfere with sexual pleasure. The degree of disability in women created by limitations of hip movement tends to be much greater than that suffered by men. Limitations in the ability of a woman to move the hip bone, especially if it is two-sided, may prevent penetration by the man. There are usually alternative positions that can be utilized. For most women, rear entry positions are still possible despite hip disease. Fortunately, hip problems in men are unlikely to interfere significantly with the mechanical performance of sexual intercourse.

Sufficient preparation for intercourse may be necessary for patients with the most severe back and arthritic problems. Many need a warm-up period similar to that utilized by athletes. Such people may need to have the application of moist warm heat to affected joints. Warm baths, showers, or compresses help to limber up joints prior to having sexual relations. Many doctors encourage arthritic patients to use such procedures as part of foreplay. When a couple bathes together before sex, they get a mutual application of moist heat. The pleasure of such an experience often enables them to forget the medicinal aspect of bathing.

The time of day used for sexual activity may affect the amount of pain experienced. Many patients with osteoarthritis prefer mornings. In rheumatoid arthritis patients, fatigue tends to decrease just before noon and again in mid-afternoon. The majority of patients with arthritis have less stiffness at night, making that the best time for sexual intercourse.

A complete and candid discussion of sexual problems with the patient's doctor is absolutely essential. Until that is accomplished, a person should not decide that sexual intercourse is impossible, whatever the physical handicap. Furthermore, if sexual intercourse is mechanically impossible, the doctor may discuss alternative means of obtaining sexual gratification. The real goal of sexual activity is the interpersonal pleasure and the intimacy it can bring to a relationship. There are many alternative methods of sexual gratification that can be utilized, even when sexual intercourse is not physically practical. Such methods include masturbation, fellatio (oral sexual stimulation of the penis) and cunnilingus (oral sexual stimulation of the female genitalia).

Fortunately, however, most backache patients can utilize varying techniques to successfully engage in and enjoy sexual intercourse. Most men with low back problems can engage in intercourse lying flat on the back, utilizing the position of the man below and the woman above. At other times, the side-to-side position enables normal relations. A woman with low back problems may discover she can have pain-free intercourse by lying flat on her back with her knees supported by a pillow, and straddled by the man in a superior position. Alternatively, the woman can be on her back or side with one leg raised enabling the man to make a side penetration. In another variation, the woman can be standing, leaning over a table or bed, allowing the man to make a rear penetration. All these may be comfortable and satisfying positions for women with severe back problems.

Patients should inquire of their doctors about positions for intercourse that are most adaptable for their affected joints. Through their own experience, some people will discover workable positions and such trials should be encouraged. Usually, the doctor can recommend positions, such as those just described, that take weight off painful joints. It is also helpful for people to be reassured by their doctors that unfamiliar sexual practices may simply be normal variations and not perversions.

In the past, patients suffering from chronic pain, such as the pain of arthritis, have indicated to their doctors that they felt sexual activity made them feel better. Some even said that the sexual act relieved their pain. Because of this, studies have been conducted to discern the action of sexual activity in chronic pain patients. A recent study was conducted with arthritis patients, all of whom were sexually active. It revealed that their sexual activity not only made these patients feel better, but it also relieved their pain. It is unclear whether the sexual activity, in itself, functions as an analgesic. It may well be that the pain is still there, but after a positive sexual experience, it just does not bother the person quite so much.

If a backache problem intensifies, or in other ways becomes disturbing during sexual activity, auto-acupressure may provide the solution. Auto-acupressure can ordinarily be utilized during sexual relations to relieve, or eliminate, backache without disturbing the natural flow of events. Whatever the technique or method being employed, most people can usually find a way to free one or both hands for the brief time necessary to produce backache relief. Even if the affected person cannot (for whatever psychological or physical reasons) bring himself (or herself) to utilize auto-acupressure during sexual activities, there are still many alternative methods to obtain relief from backache, utilizing the auto-acupressure systems.

The sexual partner can apply pressure either to the auto-acupressure body system or ear system of points. Either sexual partner can perform, or assist with, the brief application of a transcutaneous neurostimulator on an auto-acupressure system body point. Patients have reported that brief stimulation of a body system point with a vibrator (that can be used for genital stimulation) not only relieved their backache, but also made their overall sexual experience more pleasurable.

Unfortunately, some readers may want to disregard the advice given in this chapter. Such will be the fate of those who suffer backache, and use that difficulty as an excuse for avoiding sexuality. Such people do exist. Pain problems are used for avoiding responsibilities and intimacy. Such avoidance techniques are the equivalent of statements used humorously, in common parlance, to describe the effect of pain on the ability to perform. The statement, 'Not tonight dear, I have a backache,' has meaningful connotations. Readers of this chapter may be either burdened or relieved to know that their chronic pain problems need *not* be a replacement for a fulfilling sexual life.

Epilogue
SOME PARTING ADVICE

Not long ago, I was rushing through the radiology department of the university hospital where I practise. I caught up to a colleague who specializes in cardiology, and we exchanged greetings. He then made a rather serious indictment of himself, which unfortunately applied even more accurately to me.

'I never cease to be astonished at the amount of sensible advice—about reducing their workload—that I give to my patients,' he emphasized with remorse, 'but that I totally disregard myself.'

Although daily pressure and fatigue are not unique to the practice of medicine, I contemplated the rigours of having a conference scheduled at seven-thirty that morning and a staff meeting scheduled to last after nine that night. The intervening hours were to be overloaded with work. There would be patients scattered over numerous hospital wards, medical students and residents needing guidance, other medical specialists depending on my expertise as I depend on theirs, an office filled with harried people in distress, and an insatiable telephone. Hours full of pressure, of major and minor decisions, of facilitating health and relieving pain, of struggling to improve the quality and quantity of life.

Quite candidly, auto-acupressure provides the pain relief which enables me to work that hectic schedule. Moreover, auto-acupressure is effective for my patients and also for my readers. Their letters of appreciation fill my filing cabinets.

As I complete this epilogue in September 1979, I would like to share the contents of a letter which arrived this week. An attorney living in a distant state chronicled his battle with a pain problem, which lasted for half a dozen years prior to acquiring my first book on auto-acupressure. He hoped that the promise of quick pain relief without drugs 'might actually be realizable'. He concluded:

> In 1977, I read about your book, bought it, read it and applied its principles. It works! The need for the 'treatment' became less and less frequent and now a couple of weeks and more go by between symptoms. Upon auto-acupressure, they disappear in short order.
>
> Your book has helped me tremendously and the virtual absence of pain has rekindled my enthusiasm for work. I am sure it has helped others—undoubtedly a lot more than you have heard from.

I must stress again that auto-acupressure for backaches is a medical, not a magical, technique. Many have felt that auto-acupressure has helped them recover from pain-related disabilities and enhanced their joy of life.

I hope you will share that experience.

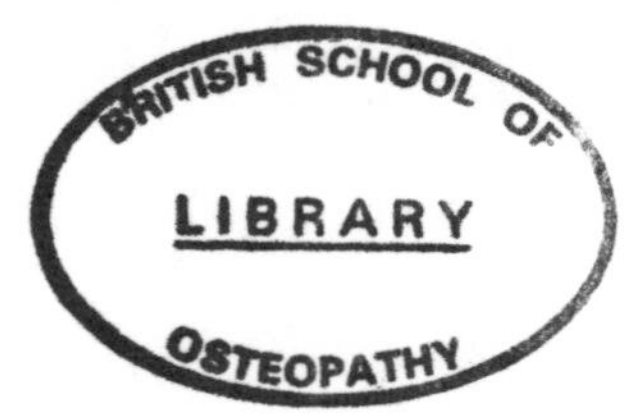

INDEX

Index